## DATE DUE

| MAR 0 7 1994 | |
|---|---|
| | |
| | |
| | |
| | |
| | |
| | |
| | |
| | |
| | |
| | |
| | |
| | |
| | |
| | |
| | |
| | |
| GAYLORD | PRINTED IN U.S.A. |

# THE HEALING AND
# SCARRING OF
# ATHEROMA

# ADVANCES IN EXPERIMENTAL MEDICINE AND BIOLOGY

# THE HEALING AND SCARRING OF ATHEROMA

Edited by

## Moshe Wolman
Sackler School of Medicine
Tel Aviv University
Tel Aviv, Israel

PLENUM PRESS • NEW YORK AND LONDON

Library of Congress Cataloging in Publication Data

World Association of Societies of Pathology (Anatomic and Clinical). World Congress
  (11th: 1981: Jerusalem)
  The healing and scarring of atheroma.

  (Advances in experimental medicine and biology; v. 168)
  "Proceedings of the Eleventh Triennial World Congress of pathology held in late
1981 in Jerusalem, Israel."
  Bibliography: p.
  Includes index.
  1. Atherosclerosis—Congresses. I. Wolman, Moshe, 1914–      . II. Title. III.
Title: Atheroma. IV. Series. [DNLM: 1. Arteriosclerosis—Complications—Congresses.
W1 AD559 v. 168 / WG 550 H434 1981]
  RC692.W68   1981                   616.1′36                   83-24562
  ISBN 0-306-41514-3

Proceedings of the Eleventh Triennial World Congress of Pathology
held in late 1981 in Jerusalem, Israel

©1984 Plenum Press, New York
A Division of Plenum Publishing Corporation
233 Spring Street, New York, N.Y. 10013

Printed in the United States of America

The study of atherosclerosis centered since the first decade of the present century on etiology and pathogenesis. In fact, the studies of the military academy of medicine in St. Petersburg have opened the way of inducing atherosclerosis in animals. Pathogenesis of atheroma has been studied since then in humans and animals naturally prone to the development of the disease and by a variety of dietary and other procedures. The various experimental studies allowed science to evaluate the relative importance of different factors (genetic, dietary, hormonal, pharmacological, mechanical, circulatory, etc.) in atherogenesis.

Epidemiological studies as well as biochemical plasma lipid and lipoprotein estimations coupled with light microscopic, histochemical and electron microscopic investigations decreased the gap between observations on the human and experimental animal research. The enormous literature covering this field allows the intelligent reader to formulate a comprehensive concept regarding etiological factors and pathogenesis of atherosclerosis. Its impact on preventive and curative medicine was however limited in scope.

Study of atherosclerosis, the chief killer of adequately-fed populations, is of primary interest to physicians whose job is to prevent and treat illnesses. Thus, although theoretical considerations are of great interest and importance for a variety of reasons the main reason why humanity spends so much energy and money on the study of atherosclerosis is practical. The medical (including the scientific-medical) community, whose job it is to do its utmost to prevent or minimize the functional deficits, sufferings and mortality caused by atherosclerosis, is likely to pose the following questions at the head of its list of pressing problems:

1.  Can atherosclerosis be prevented and by what means?
2.  Can established atherosclerosis stop its progress, and can it regress?
3.  Can regression, healing and/or scarring be of clinical significance in improving the perfusion of organs supplied by the involved arteries?

It is obvious that perfusion of organs depends, as far as the
arteries are concerned, on two factors: elasticity of the vessel
wall and the size of its cross section areas.  The elastic properties of arteries are greatly deranged by the atherosclerotic process in all its phases and mainly in the stage of scarring or calcification.  Elasticity of the arterial wall plays a minor role in the
clinical phenomena in comparison to the effect of narrowing of the
lumen.  A major problem is, therefore, that of the effect of healing
of the atherosclerotic process on organ perfusion.

Healing by scarring associated with marked contraction of the
vessel will obviously not be beneficial for organ perfusion.
Restitutio ad integrum or healing without reduction in size of the
arterial lumen are the goals which scientists are trying to reach.
Some attempts at reaching these aims, their limitations and inherent
difficulties are reported in this book.

Answers to these questions, however temporary and partial, are
of cardinal importance.  Medical scientists and practitioners are
entitled to compact, understandable and, if possible, clinically
applicable answers to these questions.  It is the purpose of this
small book to supply up to date knowledge regarding these points.
The book is based on a symposium held within the framework of the
Eleventh Triennial World Congress of Pathology in Jerusalem in
late 1981.

Moshe Wolman, M.D.
Chairman, Department of Pathology
Tel Aviv University Sackler School of Medicine
Tel Aviv, Israel

CONTENTS

# PATHOLOGICAL PRINCIPLES INVOLVED IN REGRESSION OF ATHEROSCLEROSIS

C.W.M. ADAMS

Department of Pathology
Guy's Hospital Medical School
St. Thomas's Street
London SE1 9RT
U.K.

## SUMMARY

The view is advanced that regression of atherosclerosis depends on normal pathological principles,
namely the process of organization. On account of the
hypoxic milieu of the arterial wall and lack of capillary
ingrowths into it, the hypoxia-resistant arterial smooth
muscle cell subserves the functions of both phagocyte
and fibroblast in organization. The proliferation of
smooth muscle in atherosclerosis is, thus, attributed
to a variant of a basic pathological mechanism, and
does not require more a complex explanation, such as
the action of a somatotropin, mitogen or mutagen.
Moderate dilatation of the arterial wall, caused by the
basic pathological mechanisms of either atrophy or hypertrophy would, within definite limits, offset inward
encroachment by atherosclerosis and, thus, could
constitute another type of regression, or at least a
failure of lumen calibre to get worse.

Repair is a term that has been little used in the research literature on atherosclerosis. Previously some attention was given to the process by Gilmann (1969) in his long-continued work on regeneration and remodelling of the vasculature in the pregnant puerperal uterus. Recently the term regression has been applied to any amelioration of atherosclerosis, but it is not at all clear exactly what this term means.

In some species the lipid in experimental athero-sclerosis is largely removed after return to a fat-free or low-fat diet (e.g. Armstrong and Megan 1972; Vesselinovitch et al., 1976). In other species, there is little or no removal of lipid (summarized by Adams and Morgan, 1977). Removal of fibrous tissue from experimental atherosclerotic lesions seems to be minimal Radhakrishnamurthy et al., 1975) and, in fact, it may increase (e.g. Antischkow 1933). Collagen types vary during atherogenesis (McCullagh and Balian, 1975) and subsequent "regression", and this seems to be associated with an active phase of collagen synthesis and then reunion to a mature collagen type.

Although hallowed by some years' use, regression is not the best of terms, as we are not distinguishing between lipid removal, collagen turnover and resorption, and progressive age-wise dilatation of the arterial wall (Wilson et al.,1978). Moreover, neither of the first two events necessarily implies any clinical change. It is only increase of the arterial lumen that would result in a practical clinical benefit.

Although the term regression seems to be with us, it has another unfortunate result in that it confuses or ignores the pathological principles that are involved. The position is really exceedingly simple. Athero-sclerosis may heal, to a greater or lesser extent, by the general pathological process known as organisation. As is well known to a first year medical and as shown in the last century by Cohnheim (1889), organisation proceeds by three phases:-

(a)    invasion or entry of capillary sprouts, derived from endothelial cells
(b)    phagocytosis of debris, normally by blood-derived mononuclear phagocytes (monocytes becoming macro-phages)
(c)    structural repair by collagen, normally synthesized by fibroblasts.

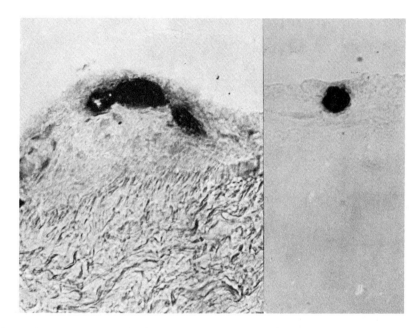

Fig. 1.   Subendothelial position of mononuclear
          phagocytes (blood monocytes) in small fibrous
          atherosclerotic lesion and in normal human
          aortic wall.  Cytochrome oxidase, x 400.
          Figs. 1 and 3-6 are reproduced by permission
          of the editor of Atherosclerosis.
          (Reduced 10% for reproduction.)

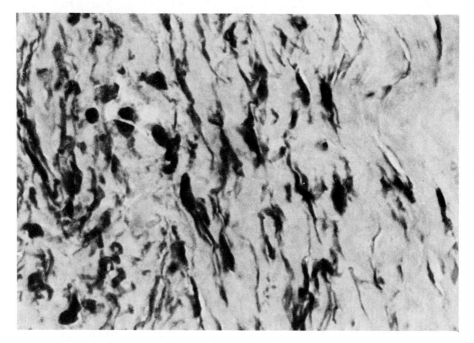

Fig. 2.    Smooth muscle in deeper parts of fibrofatty
           atherosclerotic plaque in human aorta.
           Modified Gomori trichrome, x 300.
           (Reduced 10% for reproduction.)

It is the purpose of this paper to consider how effective is the basic pathological process of organization in 'regression' of atherosclerosis, and to what extent is it modified. The ingrowth of capillary sprouts into the area to be repaired is obviously essential in repair to allow (a) ingress of mononuclear phagocytes and (b) to provide adequate oxygen for the haloperoxide-dependent process of phagocytosis. However, it is a peculiar feature of the normal arterial wall (shared with the tendon and cornea) to be avascular, and to rely on direct permeation of oxygen and nutriments from the lumen (Kirk and Lausen,1955; Heughen et al., 1973). Where the vessel wall exceeds a certain thickness, as in the aorta, part is nourished by vasa vasorum that penetrate there from the adventitia (Woerner, 1959; Wolinsky and Glagov,1967). The inner part of the vessel wall, i.e. that principally involved in atherosclerosis, is still nourished by permeation from the lumen. This avascular nature of the arterial wall would discourage monocyte entry, as can be shown by the failure of mononuclear phagocytes to penetrate deep into the human arterial wall (fig 1; Adams et al., 1975; Gaton and Wolman, 1977). This failure of monocytes to enter at depth is no doubt the explanation for the numerous fat-filled smooth muscle cells to be seen in human atherosclerotic lesions (fig. 2) or, in other words, vascular smooth muscle acts here as a phagocytic cell because the regular phagocytic cell is unable to survive under these hypoxic conditions.

The third feature of organization is the laying down of collagen or fibrous tissue, and this function is also taken over by arterial smooth muscle (Ross and Klebanoff, 1971) and typical fibroblasts are absent. Again the fibroblast presumably requires a vascular supply of capillary sprouts. One might ask how it is that arterial smooth muscle cells survive in the hypoxic intima and inner media. The answer would seem to be that arterial smooth muscle can readily respire anaerobically (see Lehninger, 1959). Indeed, arterial and venous smooth muscle show no succinic dehydrogenase detectable by histochemical methods, in contrast to the strong reaction of intestinal and ureteric smooth muscle (Adams and Bayliss, 1976). However, the capacity of arterial smooth muscle to revert to aerobic metabolism (Pasteur brake) may be greater than at first thought.

The upshot of these considerations is that the process of organisation in atherosclerosis is mediated

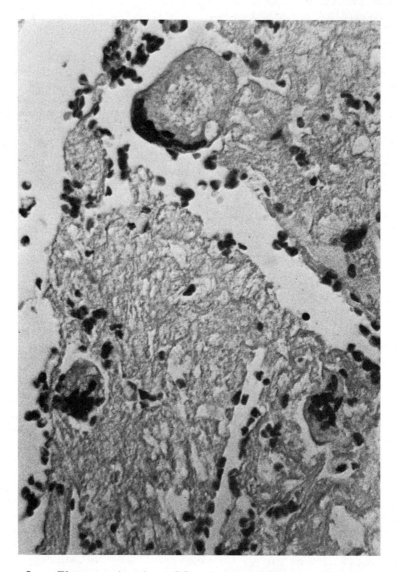

Fig. 3.  Three giant cells in capillarized advanced
         human aortic atherosclerotic plaque.
         Haematoxylin and eosin, x 400.
         (Reduced 10% for reproduction.)

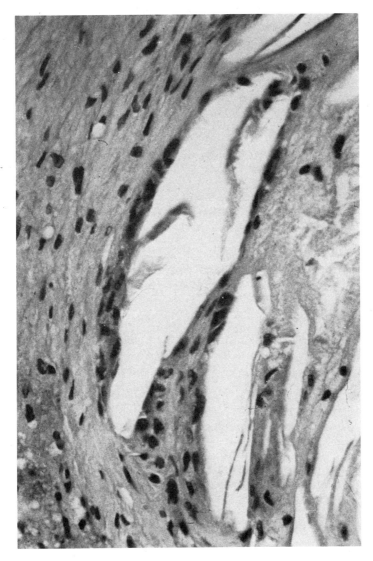

Fig. 4. Mononuclear phagocytes pallisaded round a cholesterol cleft in advanced human aortic atherosclerosis. Haematoxylin and eosin, x 400. (Reduced 10% for reproduction.)

largely by arterial smooth muscle, and not by mononuclear
phagocytes and fibroblasts.   This preference is dictated
by the essential absence of capillaries in the arterial
wall and in uncomplicated atherosclerotic lesions.
However, the further development of atherosclerosis,
with the complications of ulceration, mural thrombosis,
haemorrhage etc., leads to an incursive blood supply.
Under these circumstances, macrophages may then enter
the arterial wall (Adams and Bayliss,1976) leading to
the occasional formation of macrophage-derived giant
cells (fig. 3); particularly around cholesterol clefts
(fig. 4; Bayliss-High and Adams, 1980).

    The role of smooth muscle proliferation in athero-
sclerosis is then not such a mysterious event.   There
is no need to invoke new concepts of somatotropin (Ross
et al., 1974), mitogen or a mutagen (Benditt, 1974).
Arterial smooth muscle would now appear as a hypoxia-
resistant mesenchyme cell which, faut mieux, takes over
the functions of mononuclear phagocyte and fibroblast
(see fig. 2).   The former function is inefficient and
perhaps explains why lipids so readily accumulate in
atherosclerotic lesions.   The latter function accounts
for the fibrous cap over the typical atherosclerotic
lesion.

    Organization follows the process of inflammation,
particularly where the inflammation is chronic or where
there is substantial loss of tissue.   There is undoubtedly
an inflammatory element in atherosclerosis, and this may
result from mechanical haemodynamic damage to the wall
(Virchow, 1856), from the irritant even necrotizing
effects of certain sterols (Baranowski et al., 1982),
from fibrin encrustation (Duguid, 1948) and, possibly,
as a result of an immune reaction, as suggested by the
frequent lymphocyte accumulations seen in the tunica
adventitia in severe atherosclerosis.   Although, the last
is perhaps more of a response than a primary mechanism,
and is perhaps an autoimmune event, yet the other factors
could well operate from an early stage in the development
of atherosclerosis.   Diffuse intimal thickening (Geer and
Haust, 1972) and the musculo-elastic hyperplastic layers
(Morgan, 1956) may result more from reparative hyperplasia than from post inflammatory organisation.   In all
these reparative responses, it is the smooth muscle cell
that is mainly involved, for the reasons set out above.

    Another pathological mechanism, which is relevant
to regression, is the process of atrophy.   Age dependent

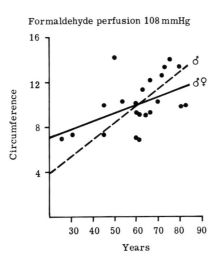

Fig. 5.  Relationship between size of coronary artery
         lumen and age.  Hearts were pressure fixed at
         mean normal blood pressure (108 mm Hg).

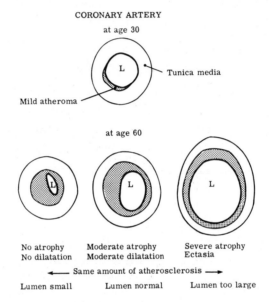

Fig. 6.   Diagram to show effect of dilatation of arterial
          wall on size of lumen, and how dilatation may
          compensate for atherosclerotic stenosis (lower
          middle).  Over dilatation (ectasia; lower
          right) results in thrombosis because of the
          distortion of local blood flow.

atrophy of the musculo-elastic elements of the wall leads
to dilatation (fig. 5) or, in severe form, ectasia
(Aschoff, 1924). Coronary ectasia is dangerous in that
it leads to too large a lumen (fig. 6 bottom right), a
reduced flow velocity, haemodynamic disturbances and the
risk of thrombosis (Wilson et al., 1978). However,
coronary dilation that keeps pace with the inward
encroachment of atherosclerosis (fig. 6 bottom centre)
can only have a beneficial effect, and would in effect
result in regression or at least a state of non-
progression (see Duguid, 1926; Adams, 1964; Wilson et
al., 1978). Dilatation is in no sense repair, yet it
contributes to the process of regression. Dilatation
can also result from hypertrophy in that the coronary
arteries can respond to increased demands by the heart
in hypertension by increasing their calibre and lumen
sizes (Harrison and Wood, 1949). Whether exercise is
also capable of leading to controlled coronary dilatation
remains to be resolved.

REFERENCES

Adams, C.W.M. 1964, Arteriosclerosis in man, other
    mammals and birds. Biol. Revs. 39, 372.
Adams, C.W.M. and Bayliss, O.B., 1976a, Detection of
    macrophages in atherosclerotic lesions with
    cytochrome oxidase. Brit. J. Exp. Pathol., 57,
    30-36.
Adams, C.W.M. and Bayliss, O.B. 1976b. Succinic
    dehydrogenase and cytochrome oxidase in arterial
    venous and other smooth muscle. Atherosclerosis,
    23, 367-370.
Adams, C.W.M. and Morgan, R.S., 1977, Regression of
    atheroma in the rabbit. Atherosclerosis, 28,
    399-404.
Adams, C.W.M., Bayliss, O.B. and Turner, D.R. 1975,
    Phagocytes, lipid-removal and regression of atheroma.
    J. Pathol., 116, 225-238.
Anitschkow, N., 1933, Experimental arteriosclerosis in
    animals, in: "Arteriosclerosis" ed. by E.V. Cowdry,
    Macmillan, London and New York.
Armstrong, J.L. and Megan, M.B., 1972, Lipid depletion
    in atheromatous coronary arteries in rhesus
    monkeys after regression diets. Circulation 30,
    675-680.
Aschoff, L. 1924, Lectures in Pathology. Hoeber,
    New York, pp 131-153.

Baranowski, A., Adams, C.W.M., Bayliss High, O.B. and
    Bowyer, D., 1982, Connective tissue responses to
    oxysterols. Atherosclerosis, in press.
Bayliss High, O.B., and Adams, C.W.M., 1980, The role of
    macrophages and giant cells in advanced human
    atherosclerosis. Atherosclerosis, 36, 441-447.
Benditt, E.P. 1974, Evidence for the monoclonal origin
    of human atherosclerotic plaques and some
    implications. Circulation, 50, 650.
Cohnheim, J. 1889, Inflammation, in: "Lectures on
    General Pathology". The New Sydenham Society,
    London. Vol. 1. pp 242-382.
Duguid, J.B., 1926, Atheroma of the aorta. J. Path.,
    Bact. 29, 371.
Duguid, J.B., 1948, Thrombosis as a factor in the
    pathogenesis of aortic atherosclerosis. J. Path.
    Bact. 58, 207.
Gaton, E. and Wolman, M., 1977, The role of smooth
    muscle cells and haematogenous macrophages in
    atheroma. J. Pathol., 123, 123-128.
Geer, J.C. and Haust, M.D., 1972, Smooth muscle cells
    in atherosclerosis. Monographs on Atherosclerosis,
    No. 2. Karger, Basel, p. 39.
Gilmann, T., 1964, A plea for arterial biology as a
    basis for understanding arterial disease, in:
    "Biological Aspects of Occlusive Vascular Disease."
    Ed. by D.G. Chalmers and G.A. Gresham, Cambridge
    University Press, London, pp 3-23.
Harrison, C.V. and Wood, P., 1949, Hypertensive and
    ischaemic heart disease: a comparative and
    pathological study. Brit. Heart J. 11: 205.
Heughen, C., Niinikoski, J. and Hunt, T.K., 1973,
    Oxygen tensions in lesions of experimental athero-
    sclerosis in rabbits. Atherosclerosis, 17, 361.
Kirk, J.E. and Lausen, T.J.S., 1955, Diffusion
    coefficients of various solutes for human aortic
    tissue, with special reference to variation in
    tissue permeability with age. J. Gerontol., 10,
    288-302.
Lehninger, A.L., 1959, The metabolism of the arterial
    wall, in:- "The Arterial Wall" ed. by A.I. Lansing,
    Williams, and Wilkins, Baltimore, pp 220-246.
McCullagh, K.G. and Balian, G., 1975, Collagen
    characterisation and cell transformation in human
    atherosclerosis. Nature (Lond.), 258, 73.
Morgan, A.D. 1956, The Pathogensis of Coronary Occlusion,
    Blackwell, Oxford, pp 68-117.

Radhakrishnamurthy, B., Eggen, D.A., Kokatnur, Y.,
     Jirge, S., Strong, J.P. and Berenson, G.S., 1975,
     Composition of connective tissue in aortas from
     rhesus monkeys during regression of diet induced
     fatty streaks.  Lab. Invest. 33, 136-146.
Ross, R., Glomset, J., Kariya, B. and Harker, L., 1974,
     A platelet dependent serum factor that stimulates
     the proliferation of arterial smooth muscle cells
     in vitro.  Proc. Nat. Acad. Sci., 71, 1207-1210.
Ross, R. and Klebanoff, S.J., 1971, The smooth muscle
     cell.  I.  In vivo synthesis of connective tissue
     proteins.  J. Cell. Biol. 50, 159.
Vesselinovitch, D., Wissler, R.W., Hughes, R. and
     Borensztajn, J., 1976, Revisal of advanced athero-
     sclerosis in rhesus monkeys.  Part 1.  Light
     microscopic studies.  Atherosclerosis, 23, 155-176.
Virchow, R. von., 1856, Gesammette Abhandlungen zur
     Wissenschaftlichen Medicin, Berlin, Muller,
     pp 458-521.
Wilson, J., Adams, C.W.M. and Brander, W.L., 1978,
     The antiocclusive effect of coronary dilatation
     with age.  Atherosclerosis, 29, 503.
Woerner, C.A., 1959, Vasa vasorum of arteries, their
     demonstration and distribution, in: "The Arterial
     Wall", ed. by A.I. Lansing, Williams and Wilkins,
     Baltimore, pp 1-14.
Wolinsky, H. and Glagov, S., 1967, Nature of species
     differences in the medial distribution of aortic
     vasa vasorum in mammals.  Circulat. Res. 20, 490-


ACKNOWLEDGMENT

The author is indebted to the British Heart Foundation
who supported some aspects of the work reported herein.

# MACROPHAGE ACTIVATION IN THE PREVENTION OR

# REGRESSION OF ATHEROSCLEROSIS

Edith Gaton and Moshe Wolman

Department of Pathology
Tel Aviv University, Sackler School of Medicine
Tel Aviv, Israel

## INTRODUCTION

Studies of our group, first presented at a meeting of the Israel Atherosclerosis Society in 1973, indicated that atheromatosis might be the result of imbalance between the amounts of lipids absorbed in – or synthesized by the intima and the amounts removed or metabolized. According to this notion the fate of intimal smooth muscle cells, whether they will or will not be transformed into foam cells and eventually burst with formation of a poltaceous lipoproteic mass, depends on the relationship between the lipid input and output processes. Absorption of lipids from the medium and synthesis are included here under the heading "input", while export of lipids from the tissues to the circulation as well as catabolism are included under "output".

It has been established that most of the lipids of atheroma are derived from plasma lipoproteins (Duff and McMillan, 1951; Watts, 1971; Wolinsky et al., 1975) which are endocytosed by intimal myocytes. The flow of plasma lipoproteins from the blood stream across the arterial wall has been corroborated by Sinapius (1980), who found lipid droplets apparently migrating across arterial walls. The lipids in the myocytes are subsequently found in secondary lysosomes of these cells. (Shio et al., 1974; Goldfischer et al.,1975)

---

* This study was subvented in part by grants from the Bureau of the Chief Scientist, Ministry of Health, Israel. The authors are grateful to N. Dietch, T. Eldar, D. Galmor and I. Peer for technical help, to A. Pinkasov and L. Levy for the photographic work, and to Mr. N.H. Rothschild for the animal care.

15

Thus, The input of lipids into the cells may be expected to depend
mainly on the concentration and physico-chemical state of lipids in
the extracellular compartment. The output (catabolism and export)
may be expected mainly to depend on the capacity of lysosomal enzymes
to render the stored lipids digestible or transportable. In both
pathways emulsification of the stored hydrophobic lipids probably
plays a key role by enabling the cells to deal with the absorbed
fats.

In view of the fact that genetically determined lack of acid
esterase causes in two diseases (Wolman disease and cholesterol
ester storage disease, Wolman, 1981) transformation of involved
cells into foam cells. We suggested that lack of this enzyme activity
in relation to the amounts of absorbed lipids might play a central
role in atheromatosis.

Experimental evidence adduced by our group on animals with
different tendencies to develop spontaneous and experimental
atherosclerosis (Wolman, 1974), on animals with experimental
hyperlipidemia (Gatom et al., 1975), hypertension (Gaton et al., 1976)
and aortic ligation (Michowitz et al., 1977) supported our notion.

Studies by other groups led them to formulate similar notions
(De Duve, 1974; Shio et al., 1974; Wolinsky et al., 1975; Peters,
1975; Corey and Zilversmit, 1977).

Also in vitro studies made on cultured cells adduced evidence
supporting the theory that activity of lysosomal enzymes versus lipid
uptake might play a major role in lipid accumulation and atheroma
formation (Bierman et al., 1974; Goldstein et al., 1977; Kar and
Day, 1978; Mitani et al., 1979). Recently Haley et al. (1980) found
no correlation between the amount of lipids and the intensity of
cholesteryl esterase activity in cells of aortae of rabbits with
experimental atheromatosis. The authors concluded that the findings
are contrary to the notion that enzyme deficiency might be responsible
for atherosclerosis. This conclusion is believed not to be warranted
as the authors correlated output only and not the ratio output:
input with atherogenesis. Obviously atherogenesis depends also on
the amount of lipids endocytosed by the cells.

Studies of the group of Adams in London (Adams et al., 1975;
Adams and Bayliss, 1976) and of our group (Gaton and Wolman, 1977)
indicate that other cells in addition to myocytes play a role in
atheromatosis, possibly mainly in its regression. The cells were
identifies as macrophages. We found that while the myocytes were
relatively poor in acid esterase, the cells tentatively identified
as macrophages exhibited intense enzyme activity. The studies of
Fowler et al. (1979) supported the notion of a dual nature of the
cells of atheroma and the studies of Yatsu et al. (1980) and of
Schaffner et al. (1980) indicated that the level of lysosomal

esterase in macrophages plays an important role in atherogenesis and possibly also in regression of the lesions.

The various studies mentioned above used different technics to demonstrate the lipolytic activity of lysosomes on the different cells. While the studies of some groups, including ours utilized an acyl esterase technic, other groups measured cholesteryl esterase activity. It is important, therefore, to establish the nature of the enzyme the lack of which is presumed to be responsible for lipid storage in myocytes and which is present in macrophages. The question is closely related to that of the nature of the enzyme deficiency in Wolman disease and of the nature of the lipolytic enzymes in the lysosomes of macrophages.

In Wolman disease and cholesterol ester storage disease lack of an enzyme demonstrable by an acyl esterase technic was found to be the main pathogenic factor. Although a single biochemical and histochemical technic does not necessarily indicate the presence of one enzyme, it is probable that the genetic disturbance affects a single enzyme which is capable of hydrolysing both long and short chain acyl esters as well as cholesteryl esters. This reasoning is not necessarily valid for normal tissues in which different enzymes might play a role in lipolytic activities (Severson and Fletcher, 1978; Mitani et al., 1979). The liver was reported in fact to contain at least 10 different fractions exhibiting acid esterase activity (Markert and Hunter, 1959).

Acid lipase, acyl esterase and cholesteryl esterase were studied by many authors as distinct enzymes. Brecher et al. (1978) on the other hand, found that the aorta of rabbits contains a single esterase capable of splitting the different substrates. Similar findings were obtained by Brown and Sgoutas (1980) in the rat liver enzyme.

The above data obtained by our group and others prompted us to formulate the following working hypothesis:

While the appearance of intimal foam cells depends on the "input:output" ratio in the myocytes, macrophages invading the lesion from the blood stream are rich in lysosomal esterase activity and may play a role in the regression and prevention of atheroma. These enzyme-rich cells were seen in both human full-blown atheromata (Wolman, 1974; Barbey and Borit, 1976) and in those of experimental animals. Theoretically, presence of a large number of such cells in the intima might reduce the amount of lipid available for ingestion by myocytes and delay atherogenesis. At the stage of mature atheroma, macrophages might clear the lipid debris and allow healing by fibrous scarring.

Macrophages were implicated in the past in the pathogenesis of atheroma, but various studies attributed to them different roles.

On the one hand some studies (Leary, 1941; Gordon, 1947; Poole
and Florey, 1958; Gerrity, 1981 a and b) have shown that lipid-laden
macrophages can penetrate the arterial intima. This was assumed to
represent an early and important step in atherogenesis. On the other
hand other authors, for example Patek and Bernick (1960, 1961) have
shown that reticuloendothelial blockade accelerated the development
of experimental atherosclerosis in rabbits and rats.

It appears, therefore, that the reticuloendothelial system might
exert different activities which affect the development and fate of
atheromatous plaques. On the one hand, activation of phagocytic cells
might increase the amount of lipids carried in foam cells into the
arterial intima and favor atherogenesis. On the other hand, activation
of the R.E.S. might reduce the amount of lipoprotein particles (LDL)
penetrating the arterial wall. Different effects of R.E.S. activation
on atherogenesis might be related to the effects of activation of
macrophages in other processes. The effect of R.E.S. activators such
as B.C.G. (Weiss et al.,1966; Ishibashi et al.,1978) or levan (Sinai
et al.,1976) on isogeneic tumor development depends on the schedule
and timing of treatment. Activation of macrophages at a given period
inhibits tumor growth, while the same procedure performed at a
different stage enhances tumor growth. It is obvious therefore, that
study of the effect of macrophage activation must include different
time patterns of administration of the activating agents.

Furthermore, numerous studies have shown that the term
"activation" of macrophages includes a number of processes. Various
activating agents stimulate different activities (Wing et al., 1977;
Wolman and Eldar, 1981) and few data are available regarding
activation which would include activities which are presumably
needed for inhibition of atherogenesis, such as: proliferation,
swelling and spreading of cells, increased phagocytic activity as
well as increased lysosomal lipolytic activity.

Lipid or lipid-containing activators were considered to be
likely, but not necessarily the only candidates for activators which
would enhance lipolysis. Some triglycerides were shown to be effective activators of the R.E.S. (Cooper, 1964). Some stilbene compounds
and especially diethylstilbestrol were also shown to exhibit macrophage
activating effect (Nicol et al., 1958; Boorman et al., 1980) and more
recently Ravi Subbiah (1977) has shown that estrogen stimulates
cholesteryl ester hydrolysis. Our group has previously found (unpublished results) that macrophages stimulated by high molecular levan
have a markedly decreased acid esterase activity. The effect of
levamisol, another potent macrophage activator (Mariano and
Malucelli, 1980) on acid esterase does not seem to have been
previously studied. The above considerations indicate that study
of effect of R.E.S. activation on atherosclerosis must include
activating agents which exhibit different effects on macrophage
acid esterase activity.

The present studies were based on these notions and were aimed at increasing the number of enzymatically active macrophages in the intima at various stages of atherogenesis. Such attempts might involve different effects on the monocyte-macrophage population such as: 1) proliferative stimulus causing an increase in the number of active cells belonging to the reticulo-endothelial system; 2) "activation" of macrophages in the direction of increased acid esterase activity in their lysosomes; 3) "activation" of macrophages in the direction of increased acid esterase activity in their lysosomes.

Most experiments described below deal with the effect of various activators, administered at different stages of experimental atherogenesis on the development and extent of the induced atheromatosis. The experiments done on rabbits and guinea pigs fed cholesterol-containing diet also included estimation of acid esterase activity in macrophages found within the lesions. In other experiments the effect of the R.E.S. activators on the macrophage enzyme was done with peritoneal cells.

MATERIAL AND METHODS

Experiment on Rabbits

We used 70 young female rabbits, each weighing about 2500 g. The animals were divided into two groups, the one treated for 14 weeks and the other for 19 weeks.

The short-duration group comprised three untreated animals, three treated with an atherogenic diet containing 5 % cholesterol and saline injections and experimental groups of three to six animals which were fed the atherogenic diet and treated with the following different macrophage-activating agents: B.C.G., levan levamisol, diethylstilbestrol and triolein. All injections were administered i.p.

A substantial percentage of rabbits died during the treatment and the above numbers refer only to animals which survived till the end of the experiments.

In the long-duration experiment B.C.G., levan and levamisol only were used. The doses and the treatment patterns are described in Table 1.

Experiments on Guinea Pigs

Two separate experiments were done on guinea pigs. The first experiment (experiment 2 in Table 1.) was done on 70 male, young animals weighing 250 g on the average. Except for the eight untreated animals, all the others were fed 5 % cholesterol in their diet.

Table 1. Materials and Methods

| | Rabbits | | Guinea Pigs | | |
|---|---|---|---|---|---|
| | Exp 1a | Exp 1b | Exp 2a | Exp 2b | Exp 3 |
| Duration of Athero-genic Diet in Days | 98 | 133 | 44 | 163 | 70 |
| **Group I - Saline** | | | | | |
| Number of Animals | 3 | 2 | 3 | 1 | 6 |
| Dose per Injection per Animal | 5 ml | 5 ml | 1 ml | 1 ml | 2 ml |
| Days of Injection | 21,42,63,84th | 98th,126th | 23rd to 26th | 124th to 127th | 4,6,9th Before Diet |
| **Group II - B. C. G.** | | | | | |
| Number of Animals | 6 | 3 | 4 | 2 | 6 |
| Dose per Injection Per Animal | 0.1 mg | 0.1 mg | 0.1 mg | 0.1 mg | 0.1 mg |
| Days of Injection | 21,42,63,84th | 98th 126th | 26th | 126th | 4,6,9th Before Diet |
| **Group III - Levan** | | | | | |
| Number of Animals | 3 | 3 | 4 | 3 | 6 |
| Dose per Injection per Animal | 200 mg in 5 ml | 200 mg in 5 ml | 50 mg in 1 ml | 50 mg in 1 ml | 50 mg in 1 ml |
| Days of Injection | 2x week 5-12 w. | 2x week 14-18 w. | 23rd to 26th | 124th to 127th | 4,6,9th Before Diet |
| **Group IV - Levamisol** | | | | | |
| Number of Animals | 6 | 2 | 5 | 3 | 3 |
| Dose per Injection per Animal | 42 mg in 5 ml | 42 mg in 5 ml | 20 mg in 1 ml | 20 mg in 1 ml | 20 mg in 1 ml |
| Days of Injection | 21,42 63,84th | 98th,126th | 23rd to 26th | 124th to 127th | 4,6,9th Before Diet |
| **Group V - Diethyl Stilbestrol** | | | | | |
| Number of Animals | 5 | | | | |
| Dose per Injection per Animal | 15 mg daily | | | | |
| Days of Injection | 49th to 69th | | | | |
| **Group VI - Triolein** | | | | | |
| Number of Animals | 5 | | | | |
| Dose per Injection per Animal | see Note* | | | | |
| Days of Injection | 71,75,78 82,85,89 92th | | | | |
| **Group VII - Untreated** | | | | | |
| Number of Animals | 3 | 3 | 3 | 5 | 6 |

*Note :  0.04 ml of Emulsion (40 mg in 2 ml of 0.5% Tween 20)

In these animals 5 to 40 % cocoa butter was included in the
diet during the first few weeks of the experiments. A high mortality forced us to abandon the inclusion of cocoa butter in the diet.

The 70 animals were divided into two groups: a short-treatment
group was fed the atherogenic diet for six weeks and a long-treatment group kept on the diet for 23 weeks. Here too, control groups
were included: the one fed commercial chow only and the other fed
the diet and injected i.p. with saline on the same days as the
experimental animals.

The short-treatment group contained three untreated animals,
three given the diet and saline injections and groups of 4 to 5
animals fed the diet and injected with B.C.G., levan or levamisol.

The long-treatment group consisted of: five untreated animals,
one saline-treated animal and groups of 2 to 3 guinea pigs treated
with: B.C.G., levan or levamisol. Details are given in Table 1.

In view of the disappointing results obtained in the above
attempts, in a second experiment (Experiment 3) the various macrophage-activating agents were injected into guinea pigs before diet
was started.

Thirty male guinea pigs weighing 250 g were used. Six animals
were left untreated. All the others were fed chow containing 5 %
cholesterol over a period of 10 weeks. Prior to the administration
of diet the animals were given three successive injections of
macrophage-activating agents on days -9, -6, -4. The macrophage-
activating agents and their doses are given in Table 1.

In both rabbits and guinea pigs the animals were killed by
intra-venous or intracardiac air injections. Animals which died
during the treatment were excluded from the study.

The aortae were rapidly removed, freed from adventitial fat
and opened longitudinally. After a macroscopical evaluation of the
degree of atheromatosis the aortae were rolled around a small piece
of the heart and frozen in isopentane chilled with liquid nitrogen.
Cryostat sections - 10 $\mu$ thick were cut and stained for: H. and E.,
Oil red O and alpha-naphthyl acetate acid esterase (Lake, 1971).
The study of the rolled aortae permitted a comparison between similar
areas in the aortae of different animals.

In many rabbits the aortae were cut longitudinally into two
pieces (segments) and one of them was fixed in 4 % buffered formalin
and stained with H. and E. and Oil red O in order to obtain a better
morphology.

In Vitro Experiments on Macrophages

The effect of various activating agents on macrophage enzyme
activities was studied in mice and rabbits. In mice, four adult ICR
females were used per batch. The mice were injected i.p. on day 0
and again on day 5 - 6 with one of the following: a) 0.2 ml of
5 % levan; b) 1 ml of 2.5 % thioglycolate; c) B.C.G. - 0.2 mg in
0.2 ml phosphate buffer pH 7.4; d) levamisol - 0.1 mg in 0.2 ml
of buffer; e) 0.2 ml of a 0.1 % solution of diethylstilbestrol in
phosphate buffer.

On day 10 each mouse was injected i.p. with 2 ml of medium 199
containing 15 % newborn calf serum and 7 drops of heparin solution
(5000 i. u./ml) per 10 ml and the fluid was aspirated after a few
seconds. The lavage fluids of each group of animals were pooled and
cultured in Leighton tubes. After 24 hours the cultures were rinsed,
dried and stained by the Giemsa procedure after methanol fixation
and by the acid esterase procedure (as in the animal experiments).

In the experiments done on rabbit macrophages, the cells were
exposed to the different activators in vitro. The following experiment was performed 3 times with minor variations. In each experiment
a male rabbit, 2.5-3 kg in weight, was injected with 40 ml of 2.5 %
Na thioglycolate. Four days later the animal was anesthesized with
nembutal and the abdominal cavity was milked after repeated injections
of heparin-containing phosphate-buffered saline (PBS) and massage.
The lavage fluid was centrifuged for 10 minutes at 1000 rpm and the
sedimented cells were cultured in Leighton tubes in the culture
medium (medium 199 containing 15 % newborn calf serum). After 24 hrs
non-adherent cells were removed by lavage with PBS. Different cultures of adherent macrophages were then exposed for 2 hrs to the
following agents diluted 1:20 in the culture medium, except for
levamisol and diethylstilbestrol which were diluted 1:10 in the
medium. The agents used were the same as those used in the mice
experiments, except that the final concentrations of the agents were
10 - 20 times lower. The cultures were then rinsed and stained as
above.

RESULTS

Rabbits (Experiment No. 1)

In animals fed the atherogenic diet and injected with saline,
atheromata, in different stages of development were apparent already
after 14 weeks of treatment. Advanced atheromata could be detected
by macroscopic examination. Atheromata were most obvious in the
thoracic aorta, but their extent could be best gauged around the
orifices of the intercostal arteries (Fig. 1.).
Microscopically atheromata in different stages of development were
seen in H. and E. and Oil red O-stained sections. (Figs. 2-5).

In many instances the inner part of the media or occasionally most of the width of the media were studded with sudanophilic droplets situated in swollen myocytes (Fig. 6). Atheromatosis was more widespread and severe in rabbits treated for 19 weeks. In both groups few or no macrophages were seen on the surface or inside the atheromata.

As in our previous experiments (Gaton and Wolman, 1977) atheromata contained two populations of cells: one of them, mostly situated in the depth of the lesion, consisted of cells with little acid esterase activity. The other population, often situated near the surface, consisted of cells with intense enzyme activity. Figures 7 and 8 show that the deeper lying cells exhibiting little enzyme activity contain bulky masses of anisotropic lipids. This indicates that lack of acid esterase activity is associated with absent capacity of emulsifying the intracellular lipid. The cells lying near the surface (macrophages), which are rich in enzyme activity contain small amounts of well emulsified lipid. These observations confirm our previously exposed notion that macrophages can and do emulsify atheroma lipids.

Comparison of the extent of atheromatosis in the animals treated with R.E.S. activators showed that treatment with triolein, diethylstilbestrol, levamisol and B.C.G. increased the severity of the process as judged by macroscopic examination and study of H. and E. and oil red 0-stained sections. Treatment with levan had less effect on the severity of the process (Table 2.).

The number of cells other than foam cells (presumably macrophages freshly arrived from the bloodstream) within atheromata appeared to be markedly increased in all animals treated with the R.E.S. stimulants in comparison to rabbits injected with saline. Fig. 9 shows clumping of mononuclear cells on the endothelial surface at an early stage of atherogenesis. In the intramural cells presumed to be macrophages acid esterase activity was markedly increased by triolein, B.C.G., levamisol and diethylstilbestrol treatments in comparison to the saline-injected rabbits, while levan treatment caused a marked decrease in the enzyme activity.

These data represent the general trend with marked individual variations between animals.

Guinea Pigs (Experiment No. 2)

Table 2 shows that in the animals fed the diet and injected with saline no obvious macroscopical evidence of atheroma was visible after 6 or 23 weeks of treatment. Microscopically, the intima and the inner part of the media contained numerous sudanophilic droplets with early atheromatous plaques. No macrophages were seen on the surface or in the intima.

Table 2.  Effects of Stimulation of Macrophages During the Dietary Regimen

| | | Macrophage – Stimulating Agents | | | | | |
| --- | --- | --- | --- | --- | --- | --- | --- |
| | | Saline | B.C.G. | Levan | Levamisol | Diethyl Stilbestrol | Triolein |
| Rabbits Exp. 1. | Atheroma | ++ | ++++ | ++ | +++ | +++ | ++++ |
| | Sudanophilia | +++ | +++ | + | +++ | +++ | +++ |
| | Nr. of Macrophages | - | ++ | + | ++ | ++ | ++ |
| | Acid Ester Activ in Macrophages | ++ | +++ | + | ++++ | +++ | +++ |
| Guinea Pigs Exp. 2. | Atheroma | - | + | ++ | ++ | | |
| | Sudanophilia | + | + | +++ | ++ | | |
| | Nr. of Macrophages | - | +++ | ++ | + | | |
| | Acid Ester Activ in Macrophages. | - | ++ | + | +- | | |

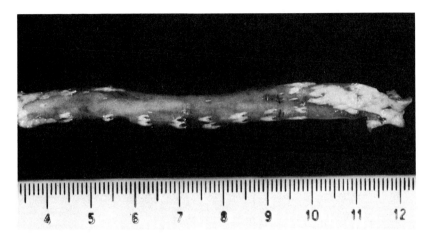

Fig. 1. Atherosclerosis in a rabbit aorta. Plaques are present
        and are best seen around the orifices of the intercostal
        arteries.

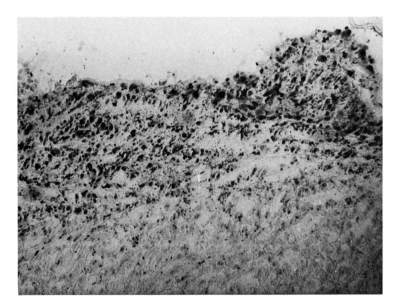

Fig. 2. An early atheromatous plaque in right upper corner bulging
        into the aortic lumen. Lipid droplets are present in the
        bulge and in the somewhat swollen intima in the upper part
        of the figure extending into the media on left center.
        Oil red O x 180.

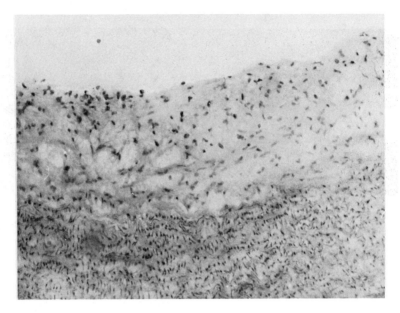

Fig. 3. Uniformly swollen intima with proliferation of cells.
Hematoxylin and eosin x 150.

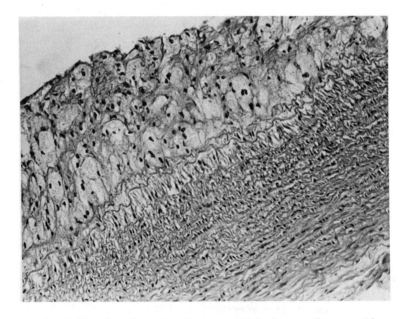

Fig. 4. Fully developed atheroma with large foam cells.
Hematoxylin and eosin x 180.

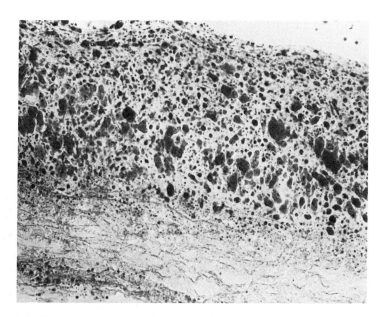

Fig. 5. A fully developed atheroma with sudanophilic lipid droplets
Oil red O x 180.

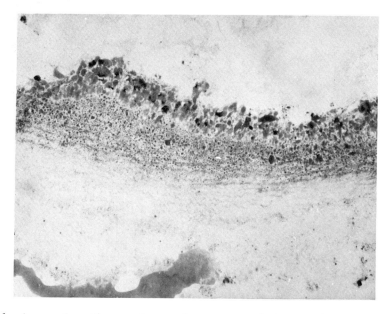

Fig. 6. An early atheromatous plaque containing weakly sudanophilic
(gray in the figure) lipoproteic droplets in the intima at the
upper part of the figure. Dark frankly sudanophilic droplets
(indicating hydrophobic lipids) in the media situated below
the intima across the figure. Oil red O x 105.

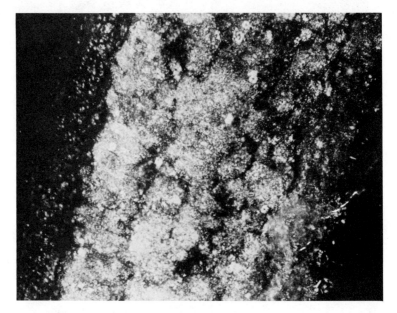

Fig. 7. Intense acid esterase activity in superficially situated
cells of an early atheroma at the left side of the figure.
Deeper areas of the intima contain cells exhibiting weak
enzyme activity. The media, on the right, shows no enzyme
activity. Alpha naphtyl acetate acid esterase x 180.

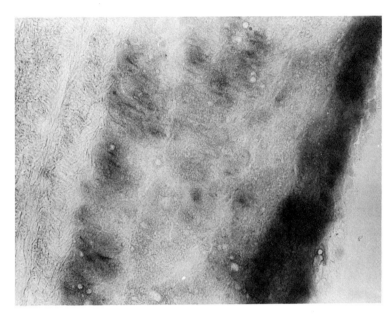

Fig. 8. The same section and field as in Fig. 7 photographed under crossed polars. Cells with intense enzyme activity on left have little lipid, while enzyme-poor areas are full of birefringent lipid droplets.

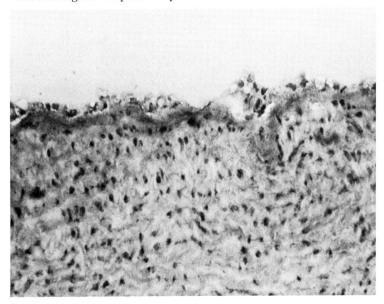

Fig. 9. Early atheroma. Monocytes and macrophages, including some foam cells lying at the luminal surface of the intima. Hematoxylin and eosin x 280.

In the levan- and levamisol- treated animals the severity of
the process was markedly increased. Frank atheromata were observed
in the aorta of most animals after both periods of treatment. The
lesions were packed with sudanophilic droplets and contained macrophages with weak acid esterase activity.

In the B.C.G.- treated guinea pigs the enhancement of atherogenesis was less pronounced than in the levan- and levamisol- treated
animals. Atheromata were smaller and the amount of sudanophilic
droplets was less. B.C.G.- treatment induced a greater number of
macrophages and a higher enzyme activity in them than in the animals
treated with the other activators.

## Guinea Pigs (Experiment No. 3)

In this experiment in which the animals were treated with
macrophage-activating agents before the diet was instituted, a
marked difference was noted between animals injected with saline
and those injected with the stimulating substances.

At the beginning of the experiment guinea pigs weighed about
250 g. Non-treated animals reached at the end of the experiment
about 700 g while the animals fed atherogenic diet and injected
with saline weighed on the average around 300 g. Guinea pigs fed
the same atherogenic diet, but injected beforehand with the different
macrophage-stimulating agents weighed at the end of the experiment
about 500 g.

The guinea pigs fed atherogenic diet and injected with saline
only appeared weak and sick. Their fur looked ruffled with yellowish
discoloration and stickiness. Some loss of hair over a dry skin was
also noted. None of these phenomena were observed in animals injected
with the macrophage-activating agents.

The aortae of animals treated with the diet and injected with
saline showed macroscopically only slight atheromatosis which was
most obvious around the intercostal vessels. Microscopically the
fatty deposits involved the intima and often the inner media.
Fig. 10  shows that levan and levamisol treatments reduced somewhat
the severity of the process, while B.C.G. almost completely inhibited
it.

It can be seen in Table 3 that the severity of atheromatosis,
as determined by microscopic criteria, was highest in guinea pigs
injected with saline and was lowest in the animals treated with
B.C.G.

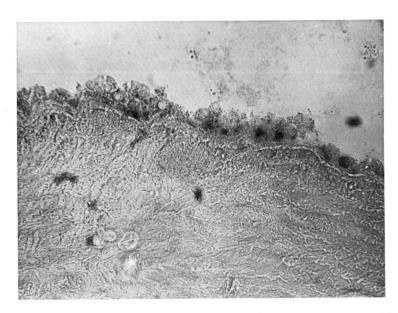

Fig. 10. Aortae of guinea pigs fed an atherogenic diet for 10 weeks.
SAL-aorta of a control animal injected i.p. with saline
shows atheromata in the thoracic part and most obviously
around the intercostal arteries. Lesser lesions are seen
in the aortae of a levan-(LN) and levamisol- pretreated (LM)
animals. The aorta on the right, of an animal pretreated
with B.C.G., is almost unaffected.

Table 3. Effects of Stimulation of Macrophages Before the Dietary
Treatment

| | | Macrophage Stimulating Agents | | | |
|---|---|---|---|---|---|
| | | Saline | B.C.G. | Levan | Levamisol |
| Guinea Pigs Exp. 3 | Atheroma | + + | − | + | − |
| | Sudanophilia | + + | ± | ± | ± |
| | Nr. of Macrophages | + + | + + | + + | + |
| | Ester Activ. in Macrophages | ± | ± | ± | ± |

Acid Esterase Activity in Isolated Macrophages

In both types of experiments in the two animal species the findings were essentially similar. On comparing only macrophages which were swollen, activated and exhibited evidence of phagocytic activity it became obvious that activation is associated in all instances with apparent loss of some acid esterase activity. This apparent loss of activity was most pronounced in macrophages exposed to levan and levamisol. With B.C.G. and to a lesser extent with the two other lipid activators (oil and diethylstilbestrol) the loss of enzyme activity was less marked.

DISCUSSION

The present experiments were based on the assumption that macrophages, which are rich in lysosomal lipolytic activity may inhibit atherogenesis and/or contribute to regression.

A number of authors (Jørgensen et al., 1972; Daoud et al., 1981) found that migration of macrophages into atheromata can be positively correlated with the intensity of damage to the vessel wall. It is reasonable to assume that the number of macrophages reaching the damaged area will depend on the size of the population from which these cells are derived and on their tendency to migrate.

We have explained in the introduction our reasons for assuming that macrophage activation might have different effects on atherogenesis in relation to the timing of administration of macrophage-activating drugs.

The results indicate that while administration of some macrophage activating agents during the feeding of atherogenic diet increased the severity of the process, partial inhibition of atherogenesis was obtained by injecting the substances before the diet. These results are surprisingly similar to those observed in the effects of macrophage activation on tumor growth mentioned in the introduction.

In the presently reported experiments the inhibition of atherogenesis was of moderate extent, probably because a single module of preventive treatment was tested and the experiment was of a rather short duration.

It is likely that variations in the schedule will result in a more effective inhibition of the process.

The different macrophage-activating substances varied in their effectiveness. It is interesting to note that B.C.G. which did not markedly decrease the intensity of acid esterase activity in macro-

phages, was also an effective antiatheromatosis agent. This fact
again strengthens our notion about the importance of acid esterase
activity in atherogenesis.

It might be permissible to speculate whether the reduction in
mortality due to coronary heart disease, observed in many countries
over the past 20 years (Stammler, 1980), might not be related to the
introduction of extensive B.C.G. vaccination. It is clear, however,
that activation of the R.E.S. by various agents might markedly change
the course of atherosclerosis.

## REFERENCES

Adams, C. W. M., and Bayliss, O. B., 1976, Detection of macrophages
      in atherosclerotic lesions with cytochrome oxidase,
      Br. J. Exp. Pathol., 57:30.
Adams, C. W. M., Knox, J., and Morgan, R. S., 1975, The resorption
      rate ot atheroma lipids in situ and implanted subcutaneously,
      Atherosclerosis, 22:79
Barbey, S., abd Borit, A., 1976, Acid esterase in human arteries,
      Histochemistry, 49:37.
Bierman, E. L., Stein, O., and Stein, Y., 1974, Lipoprotein uptake
      and metabolism by rat aortic smooth muscle cells in tissue
      culture, Circ. Res., 35:136.
Boorman, G. A., Luster, M. I., Dean, J. H., and Wilson, R. E., 1980,
      The effect of adult exposure to diethylstilbestrol in the
      mouse on macrophage function and numbers, J. Reticuloendothel.
      Soc., 28:547.
Brecher, P., Pyun, H. Y., and Chobanian, A. V., 1978, Cholesteryl
      ester and triglyceride hydrolysis by an acid lipase from
      rabbit aorta, Biochim. Biophys. Acta, 530:112.
Brown, W. J., and Sgoutas, S., 1980, Purification of rat liver
      lysosomal cholesteryl ester hydrolase, Biochim. Biophys.
      Acta, 617:305.
Cooper, G. N., 1964, Functional modification of reticulo endothelial
      cells by simple tryglicerides, J. R. E. S., 1:50.
Corey, J. E., and Zilversmit, D. B., 1977, Effect of cholesterol
      feeding on arterial lipolytic activity in the rabbit,
      Atherosclerosis, 27:201.
Daoud, A. S., Jarmolych, J., Augustyn, J. M. and Fritz, K. E., 1981,
      Sequential morphologic studies of regression of advanced
      atherosclerosis, Arch. Pathol. Lab. Med., 105:833.
De Duve, Ch., 1974, The participation of lysomomes in the transfor-
      mation of smooth muscle cells to foam cells in the aorta of
      cholesterol-fed rabbits. Acta Cardiol. (Suppl.) 20:9.
Duff, G. L., and McMillan, G. C., 1951, Pathology of atherosclerosis,
      Am. J. Med., 11:92.
Engelman, D. M., and Hillman, G. M., 1976, Molecular organization
      of the cholesteryl ester droplets in the fatty streaks of
      human aorta, J. Clin. Invest., 58:997.

Fowler, S., Shio, H., and Haley, N. J., 1979, Characterization of
    lipid-laden aortic cells from cholesterol-fed rabbits. IV.
    Investigation of macrophage-like properties of aortic cell
    populations, Lab. Invest., 41:372.
Gaton, E., Ben-Ishay, D., and Wolman, M., 1976, Experimentally
    produced hypertension and aortic esterase, Arch. Path. Lab.
    Med., 100:527.
Gaton, E., Bubis, J. J., and Wolman, M., 1975, Acid esterase in the
    aorta of the hyperlipidemic rat: A histochemical study,
    Pathol. Europ., 10:129.
Gaton, E., and Wolman, M., 1977, The role of smooth muscle cells
    and hematogenous macrophages in atheroma, J. Path., 123:123.
Gerrity, R. G., 1981 a, The role of the monocyte in atherogenesis.
    I. Transition of bloodborne monocytes into foam cells in
    fatty lesions, Am. J. Pathol., 103:181.
Gerrity, R. G., 1981 b, The role of the monocyte in atherogenesis.
    II. Migration of foam cells from atherosclerotic lesions,
    Am. J. Pathol., 103:191.
Goldfischer, S., Schiller, B., and Wolinsky, H., 1975, Lipid accum-
    ulation in smooth muscle cell lysosomes in primate atheroscle-
    rosis, Am. J. Pathol., 78:497.
Gordon, I., 1947, Mechanism of lipophage deposition in atherosclero-
    sis, Arch. Pathol., 44:247
Haley, N. J., Fowler, S., and de Duve, Ch., 1980, Lysosomal acid
    cholesteryl esterase activity in normal and lipid-laden
    aortic cells, J. Lip. Res., 21:961.
Ishibashi, T., Yamada, H., Harada, S., Harada, Y., Takamoto, M.,
    and Sugiyama, K., 1978, Inhibition and promotion of tumor
    growth by BCG: Evidence for stimulation of humoral enhancing
    factors by BCG, Int. J. Cancer, 21:67.
Jørgensen, L., Packham, M. A., Rowsell, H. C. and Mustard, J. F.,
    1972, Deposition of formed elements of blood on the intima
    and signs of intimal injury in the aorta of rabbit, pig and
    man, Lab. Invest., 27:341.
Kar, S. and Day, A. J., , 1978, Composition and metabolism of lipid
    in macrophages from normally fed and cholesterol-fed rabbits,
    Exp. Mol. Pathol., 28:65.
Lake, B. D., 1971, Histochemical detection of the enzyme deficiency
    in blood films in Wolman's disease, J. Clin. Pathol., 24:617.
Leary, T., 1941, The genesis of atherosclerosis, Arch. Path., 32:507.
Mariano, M., and Malucelli, B. E., 1980, Defective phagocytic
    ability of epithelioid cells reversed by levamisol, J. Path.,
    130:33.
Markert, C. L. and Hunter, R. L., 1959, The distribution of esterases
    in mouse tissues, J. Histochem. Cytochem., 7:42.
Michowitz, M., Gaton, E., and Wolman, M., 1977, Acid esterase
    activity in the pathogenesis of atherosclerosis: Effect of
    partial aortic ligation in rabbits, Isr. J. Med. Sci., 13:259.
Mitani, J., Suzuki, Y., Kuroiwa, T., Watanabe, Y., Kishi, Y.,

Numano, R., and Maezawa, H., 1979, Cholesterol ester hydrolase in vessel wall, Acta Histochem. Cytochem., 12:488.

Nicol, T., Bilbey, D. L. J., and Ware, C. C., 1958, Effects of various stilbene compounds on the phagocytic activity of the reticulo-endothelial system, Nature, 18:1538.

Patek, P. R., and Bernick, S., 1960, Experimental arterial lesions produced by reticuloendothelial blocking agents, A. M. A. Arch. Path., 69:35.

Patek, P. R., Bernick, S., and Frankel, H., 1961, Arterial lesions in rats by reticuloendothelial blocking agents, A. M. A. Arch. Path., 72:70.

Peters, T. Y., 1975, Lysosomes of the cardiovascular system. Progress in Cardiol., 4:151.

Poole, J. C. F., and Florey, H. W., 1958, Changes in the endothelium of the aorta and the behaviour of macrophages in experimental atheroma of rabbits, J. Path. Bact., 75:245.

Ravi Subbiah, M. T., 1977, Effect of estrogens on the activities of cholesteryl ester. 1. Synthetase and cholesteryl ester hydrolases in pigeon aorta, Steroids, 30:259.

Schaffner, T., Taylor, K., Bartucci, E. J., Fischer-Dzoga, K., Beeson, J. H., Glagov, S., and Wissler, R. W., 1980, Arterial foam cells with distinctive immunomorphologic and histochemical features of macrophages, Am. J. Pathol., 100:57.

Severson, D. L., and Fletcher, T., 1978, Characterization of cholesterol ester hydrolase activities in rabbit and guinea pig aortas, Atherosclerosis, 31:21.

Shio, H., Farquhar, M. G., and de Duve, Ch., 1974, Lysosomes of the arterial wall, Am. J. Pathol., 76:1.

Sinai, Y., Leibovici, J., and Wolman, M., 1976, Effects of route and schedule of administration of high-molecular levan on the growth of AKR lymphoma, Cancer Res., 36:1593.

Sinapius, D., 1980, Lipid deposition in the media of human coronary arteries, Atherosclerosis, 37:87.

Stamler, J., 1980, Data base on the major cardiovascular diseases in the United States, Atherosclerosis Reviews, 7:49.

Wing, E. J., Gardner, I. D., Ryning, F. W., and Remington, J. S., 1977, Dissociation of effector functions in populations of activated macrophages, Nature, 268:642.

Weiss, D. W., Donhag, R. S., and Leslie, P., 1966, Studies on the heterologous immunogenicity of a methanol-insoluble fraction of attenuated tubercle bacilli (BCG) II. Protection against tumor isografts, J. Exp. Med., 124:1039.

Watts, H. F., 1971, Basic aspects of the pathogenesis of human atherosclerosis, Hum. Pathol., 2:31.

Wolinsky, H., Goldfischer, S., Daly, M. M., Kasak, L. E., and Coltoff-Schiller, B., 1975, Arterial lysosomes and connective tissue in primate atherosclerosis and hypertension, Circ. Res., 36:553.

Wolman, M., 1974, Acid esterase as a factor in atheromatosis, Atherosclerosis, 20:217.

Wolman, M., 1981, Pathologic changes in Wolman Disease: Pathogenetic
        and possible therapeutic implications, in: Proc. 6th Int.
        Congress of Neurogenetics and Neuro-ophthalmology, Elsevier,
        North Holland, Amsterdam.
Wolman, M., and Eldar, T., 1981, Different patterns of macrophage
        activation induced by various agents, Cell. molec. Biol.
        in press.
Yatsu, F. M., Hagemenas, F. C., and Manaugh, L. C., 1980, Cholesteryl
        ester hydrolase activity in human symptomatic atherosclerosis,
        Lipids, 15:1019.

ULTRASTRUCTURAL FEATURES OF HEALING AND SCARRING OF EXPERIMENTAL

ATHEROMA

Giorgio Weber

Center of Research on Atherosclerosis - Institute of
Pathological Anatomy - University of Siena, Italy

Most of the available morphological data on regression of experimental atherosclerotic lesions of the arterial wall (rev. by
Armstrong, 1976; Wissler, 1977; Weber, 1978; Stary, 1979) have
been documented in animal models (pigs, dogs, monkeys) and are being investigated in man. It is chiefly from studies on monkeys
that our knowledge has been substantiated. Wissler et al. (1975),
Vesselinovitch et al. (1976) have demonstrated substantially reduced percentage of grossly involved aortic intima in monkeys
withdrawn from atherogenic diets. The regressing lesions contain
very little intracellular and extracellular lipid and show no evidence of a necrotic center (features that are usually prominent in
advanced atherosclerotic lesions), contain a reduced number of
cells (Stary, 1974; 1977) and are covered by an endothelial layer
of regenerating cells (Weber et al., 1977) (Fig. 1-2).
Those studies concern regression periods of 12-24 months.
Long-term regression is now being studied in great detail.
The Winston Salem Group (Clarkson et al., 1976,1979,1980; Wagner
et al., 1980a,b; Clarkson et al., 1981) working on Rhesus monkeys,
have collected a huge amount of data part of which (those concerning chemical changes) are now available. The AA. have studied
long-term regression (not only after 24 months but also after 48
months), maintaining plasma-cholesterol concentration of 300 mg/dl
or 200 mg/dl.
In the group regressed for 24 months, significantly greater
amounts of accumulated arterial cholesterol, of esterified cholesterol and phospholipid were removed in monkeys that underwent regression at 200 mg/dl of cholesterolemia in comparison to those
at 300 mg/dl. It must be noted that decreases in arterial cholesterol in the group of animals examined after 24 months at 200

37

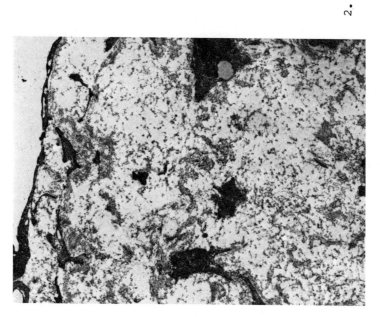

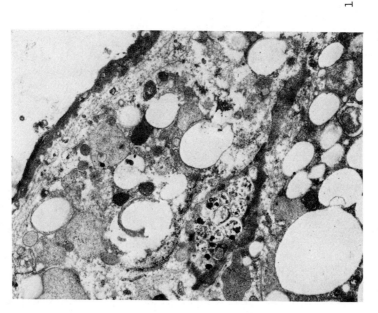

Fig. 1 – Rhesus monkey. Aorta, after 24 months on an atherogenic diet. TEM x 11.000.
Fig. 2 – Rhesus monkey. Aorta, 12 months after withdrawal from the atherogenic diet.
TEM x 9.000. (Reduced 10% for reproduction.)

mg/dl, amounted to 100% for carotid artery, 100% for thoracic aorta, 93% for abdominal aorta, 96% for iliac-femoral artery. Lesser decreases (of 80, 25, 56, 72%) were instead observed in monkeys at 300 mg/dl.

Calcified plaques were more frequent in the monkeys at higher plasma cholesterol levels. "Translated to human beings" (Wagner et al., 1980a) "these results suggest that for relatively uncomplicated fatty lesions the plasma cholesterol concentration does influence the degree of plaque regression and that greater regression may be expected to occur at plasma cholesterol concentration of 200 mg/dl as opposed to 300 mg/dl".

After 48 months of atherosclerosis regression, the monkeys had instead increased cholesterol concentration in the thoracic aorta and carotid artery (but not in abdominal aorta or iliac-femoral artery) regardless of the plasma cholesterol concentration. After regression at 300 mg/dl there was no change in frequency of calcification of the thoracic aorta while at 200 mg/dl the frequency of calcification was reduced by 50%. Increased collagen and decreased elastin content was observed in the thoracic aorta.

The AA. proposed that differences in the removal of cholesterol from thoracic and abdominal aorta after 24/48 months of regression in animals at 300 mg/dl, may be influenced by the rearranging of connective tissue.

Let us remember that also regional aortic differences in atherosclerosis susceptibility have been described by Subbiah et al. (1981) in White Carneau pigeons. Differences in regression of lesions had also been observed in mini migs: the thoracic aorta and the coronaries revealed significant reduction of cholesterol in regressing groups while no decrease was observed in the abdominal aorta (Jacobsson and Lundholm, 1981). These AA. have further informed that the effect of maintaining atherosclerotic Rhesus monkeys at plasma cholesterol concentration of 300 versus 200 mg/dl results in decreases in the mass of coronary plaques of about 30% in 4 years in the group at lower cholesterol level.

Malinow et al. (1978a,b) observed reduced size of aortic and coronary atherosclerotic lesions in Cynomolgus monkeys, still fed high cholesterol diet, if treated with cholestyramine, extending previous data in Rhesus monkeys of Wissler's Group.

Similar effects were observed in Cynomolgus monkeys fed alfa-alfa-meal (1978b).

Malinow (1981) reviewing regression studies, concludes that prolonged lowering of plasma cholesterol levels is associated with regression (removal of atheromatous materials, arrest of intimal cell proliferation, cellular repair and remodeling of the arterial wall). Furthermore, he underlines how it is yet not known the way in which changes in lipoprotein levels may trigger arterial repair processes, that nothing is known on flow in arterial lymphatics, as well as in arterial interstitial compartment and that such studies are surely needed. With the aforementioned limitations, I think

we may conclude that in non-human primates (and in other animals),
atheroregression may surely lead either to a complete disappearance of the arterial lesions (when of the "fatty streak" type) or to
a lesion thickness reduction (through cell number reduction, shrinkage or scarring) of more advanced, stenosing lesions: so leading
to a reduction also of the lumen stenosis (Stary, 1979; Malinow et
al., 1978a,b; Wissler, 1980). Regression of advanced atherosclerotic lesions in swine has been recently reviewed by Daoud et al.
(1980 and at this meeting). Regression of lesions on dogs was referred by De Palma et al. (1972).

The most recent studies insist however that regression of experimental lesions is not linear (Armstrong et al., 1980; Daoud et
al., 1980). As underlined by Clarkson et al. (1980), Wissler et al.
(1980) and Bond et al. (1981) quantitation of lesions is extremely
important and interpretation of data must be very careful.

In human pathology, observations concerning regression are
still very few (cfr. Wissler, 1978b; 1980) and chiefly developed
by Blankenhorn. He has emphasized the importance of rates of regression of lesions in volunteer subjects examined through serial arte-
riograms not only in femoral (1978) but also in coronary arteries
in 45 year old men (1980). His studies and others indicate that it
seems possible that also in our species regression of arterial lesions may take place; Thompson et al. (1978) observed regression
of atherosclerotic lesions in hypercholesterolemic patients after
plasma exchange. Olsson et al. (1981) observed with arteriographic
methods regression of atheromata in a-symptomatic, hyperlipidemic
patients subjected to hypolipidemic dietetic and pharmacological
treatment. Similar findings observed with different methodics were
also referred to by Schettler while discussing with Olsson.

Morphological (microscopic and ultrastructural) observations
are still strongly needed: it may be inferred that if in many animals the atherogenic process looks quite similar to the one developing in man, also the morphological events leading to regression
will proceed in man in a way similar to the one observed in monkeys,
even if differences both of atherogenesis and of regression in different animal models have been reported by Wissler and Vesselinovitch (1978).

Monkeys have so many advantages for studying experimental atherogenesis and atheroregression that it seems quite useless to make
use of different animal models. But for people working in Europe
the availability of monkeys is still too scarce, apart that they
are so extremely expensive and hard to care of. More available, but
still very expensive and rather hard to manage, are also swine.

For studies on atherogenesis, the rabbit model, at least in
our countries, presents some advantages indeed, the rabbits being
easily available, not too expensive, rather easy to be mana-
ged. Rabbits are moreover very susceptible to atherogenic stimuli
and quickly develop arterial lesions (Wissler and Vesselinovitch,
1974; 1978). But, in rabbits, arterial lesions are not usually con-

sidered prone to regress easily (rev. in Adams and Morgan, 1977),
unless the lesions have been induced by a short-term atherogenic
diet (Weber et al., 1975) chiefly because of cholesterol storage in
reticuloendothelial system: so that the arterial lesions, instead
of regressing, tend to progress further once one has stopped cholesterol feeding with the more prolonged periods of very high cholesterol diets (Constantinides et al., 1960). On the other hand,
Vesselinovitch et al. (1974) have been able to promote (and have
studied at gross and histologic levels) regression of aortic and
coronary lesions in rabbits subjected, after the atherogenic diet
is stopped to estrogen treatment and/or hyperoxia and cholestyramine addition to the low cholesterol regression diet. They clearly
demonstrated that regression, when helped by these additional methods, does take place also in rabbits. Wissler (1978) has summarized the available data on regression in rabbits underlining the importance of blood monocytes in phagocytosing lipids in the lesions.

We have studied aortic lesions regression in rabbits chiefly
at the ultrastructural level in an experimental condition, the partial ileal by-pass (Weber et al., 1981) developed by Buchwald et
al. (1972) also in man (Buchwald et al., 1974; Sirtori et al.,1981).
We have noted (Weber et al., 1981) that regression in rabbits has,
at ultrastructural level, many features very similar to those observed at TEM and SEM in monkeys (Stary, 1974; Weber et al., 1977).
And it cannot be disregarded here that those features of regression
are in our rabbits already evident after 30-45 days of regression
treatment: a not negligible advantage indeed of this animal model:
as accelerated models of atherogenesis and atheroregression are
needed (Lee et al., 1977).

We have observed that the hypercholesterolemia levels, which
during atherosclerosis induction could overpass the 1000 mg/dl, were
dramatically reduced after surgery to 100 mg/dl or less; a substantial reduction, up to disappearance, of gross aortic lesions
(mean intimal surface area involved from 85% to less than 12,5%),
together with a histologically relevant loss of lipid and foam
cells reduction from the residual lesions (from 73% to 39% of foam
cells). Such lesions look almost devoid of cells, while (chiefly
in the more superficial portions, but also in the deeper ones) a
deposition of matrix (elastin material, collagen and so on) is quite
evident at light and transmission EM.

At scanning EM, the lesions are no longer bulging and many of
them have almost disappeared, the continuity of the "endothelial"
layer (small regenerating cells and some monocytoid cells) appear-
ing almost completely reconstituted on them (Fig. 3-4).

In control animals, withdrawn from the hypercholesterolic
diet but not subjected to partial ileal by-pass the lesions had
not regressed at all.

The decreased cellularity observed in this experimental model
is very precocious, if compared with the one described as "drama-
tic" by Stary (1979) in primates during the "initial" period of

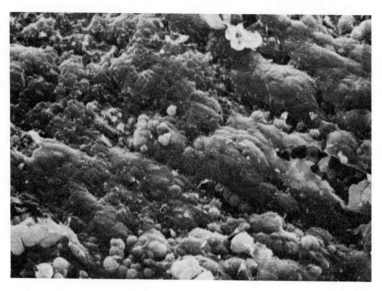

Fig. 3 - Aorta of rabbit fed a hypercholesterolic diet for 2
         months. SEM x 150.  (Reduced 10% for reproduction.)

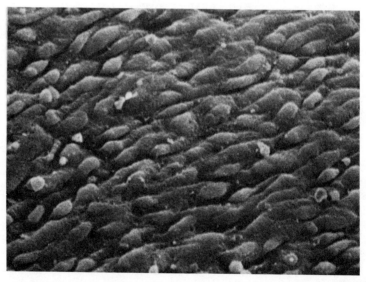

Fig. 4 - Aorta of rabbit sacrificed 45 days after withdrawal
         from the 2 months hypercholesterolic diet and the
         partial ileal by-pass intervention. SEM x 350
         (Reduced 10% for reproduction.)

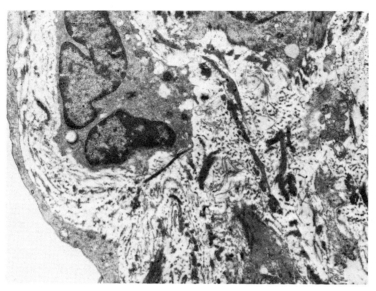

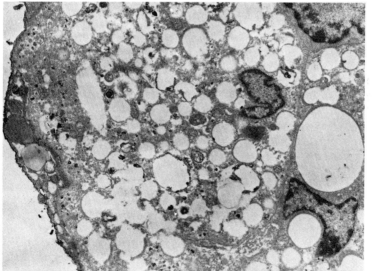

Fig. 5 – Aortic plaque of rabbit after 2 months on a hypercholesterolic diet. TEM x 4.000.
Fig. 6 – Residual aortic plaque of rabbit 45 days after withdrawal from the hypercholeste-
rolic diet and partial ileal by pass intervention. TEM x 6.500.
(Reduced 10% for reproduction.)

regression which in monkeys does correspond to 16-20 weeks of regression.

As in monkeys, also in these rabbits the lesions appear no longer fatty, but edematous, - "empty"; their outline is changed, no
more convex but flattened. Among the foam cells which are losing or
have lost the accumulated lipid, components of the matrix are increased (Fig. 5-6).

The smooth muscle cells are not perpendicularly arranged towards the lumen but are randomly or circularly disposed. Many of
them are now clearly surrounded by basement membrane (such as described by Jones et al., 1973) and some collagen (cf. Weber et al.,
1981).

We have not observed under the conditions of our study the increased numbers of lysosomes seen in the Rhesus monkeys by Stary
(1974).

It may be incidentally noted that many "foam cells" were not
easily recognizable at TEM as monocytes during regression. Instead
modified smooth muscle cells become the most prominent cells in the
regressing lesion. Therefore ultrastructural regression studies may,
when extended, help in a subsidiary way to answer the question concerning the foam cells in the lesions (rev. by Joris et al., 1979;

Over the lesions, the reconstitution of a continuous endothelial layer is evident and almost complete. The endothelial cells
may appear largely distended, but at SEM, areas may be found where
the juxtaposed cells of this "neo"-endothelial layer don't look
perfectly joined nor "flow-oriented"; in other areas, they assume
different shape and dimension; sometimes, residual lesions don't
have a continuous covering layer.

At TEM, small cuboidal juxtaposed "endothelial-like" cells
(with or without intracytoplasmatic vacuoles) are crowding and con-
stituting rows which remind the SEM pictures, where small adjacent
"plump" cells are numerous. Their Con A positive surface coat looks
simplified, almost without (or with much  less) pinocytotic vesicles; the inter-endothelial junctions usually look straight; cyto-
plasmatic organelles and Weibel-Palade bodies are conspicuous. Such
cells look in the whole less highly specialized (regenerating cells
may be functionally altered in endocytosis and possibly in proteoglycans production, Davies and Ross, 1978; Davies et al., 1980; Vlo-
dawsky et al., 1978), the area of the regressed lesions thus resulting not yet perfectly organized (Buck, 1979a, b; Christensen et
al., 1979a,b; Weber et al., 1980; Reidy and Schwartz, 1981).

While studying those features, we have been very impressed by
another finding, consisting in the presence of a well evident Con
A reactivity at the abluminal surface of the regenerating endothelial cell.

It is well known since Wight and Ross (1975) observed that the
abluminal surface of the endothelial cell does never stain with Ru-
thenium Red, nor had we ever observed a staining of this surface
with the Bernhard and Avrameas Con A reaction (1971).

It may be proposed (Weber et al., 1980) that in short-term studies (as the ones represented by these atherosclerotic rabbits) the regeneration of endothelial cells over regressing lesions is not complete. Those endothelial cells may be representing "dysfunctioning" (cfr. Gimbrone, 1980) endothelial cells. These data may help explaining the results obtained after catheter ballooning of aorta by Minick et al. (1977).

In monkeys after longer-term regression studies the endothelial regeneration reaches a more complete level (Weber et al.,1977) even if areas covered with "incompletely" regenerated endothelial cells may be still evident. Species differences are however quite different in the body of the regressing lesions: in the monkeys the matrix is extremely edematous and/or fibrous: in the rabbits, instead, the residual lesions are very impressive because of the abundant production of neo-elastic tissue which may appear ordered in rows of fragments among the smooth muscle cells which have lost most of their lipid content or may even produce a thick neo-elastic layer which runs almost parallel to the internal elastic lamina. Morphologically elastic fiber content of regressing lesions is not usually studied (cfr. Chakravarti et al., 1977). An excellent review on the topic "Connective tissue in regression" (chiefly studied biochemically) has been issued by Armstrong (1978). It may be noted that no data were available to the Author as for regressing lesions in rabbits, the only data collected concerning monkeys both for collagen and elastin which increase during atherogenesis, decrease during regression: while collagen does never return to control values elastin should even reach lower levels during regression. Observation on degradation of collagen fibers by intimal smooth muscle cells in regressing cholesterol atherosclerosis in rabbits are reported by Jurukova (1980). She has described phagocytosis of collagen fibers from part of the proliferated smooth muscle cells. Blood derived foam cells of regressing atherosclerotic lesions never displayed collagen inclusions in their cytoplasm.

Summarizing, the experimental model studied by us in rabbits, may be considered practically almost equivalent to the ones in monkeys in producing a shrinkage of lesions, which results in significant volume-decrease of the lesions and consequently of the lumen stenosis. We think, in agreement with recent statements by Wissler (1980) and Stary (1979) that lumen stenosis reduction may represent indeed a very important aim of this kind of studies, being generally agreed that growing stenosis may easily be leading to ischemic parenchymal lesions.

Our present work also confirms that, in rabbits, "atherosclerosis is a substantially reversible process" (Wissler, 1978).

But as the endothelial-like layer covering residual or regressed lesions may show signs of minor specialized ultrastructural organization, which could be signs also of minor functional capacity, our next problem is no longer to affirm or deny regression of wall-lesion but to ascertain if and when the neo-endothelial layer will result in the same functional properties of the pre-existing one.

REFERENCES

Adams, C.W.M. and Morgan, R.S., 1977, Regression of atheroma in the
    rabbit, Atherosclerosis, 28: 399.
Armstrong, M.L., 1976, Regression of atherosclerosis, Atheroscler.
    Rev., 1: 137.
Armstrong, M.L., 1978, Connective tissue in regression, Atheroscler.
    Rev., 3: 147.
Armstrong, M.L., Peterson, R.E., Hoak, J.C., Megan, M.B., Cheng, F.
    H. and Clarke, W.R., 1980, Arterial platelet accumulation in
    experimental hypercholesterolemia, Atherosclerosis, 36: 89.
Bernhard, W. and Avrameas, S., 1971, Ultrastructural visualization
    of cellular carbohydrate components by means of Concanavalin
    A, Exp. Cell Res., 64: 232.
Blankenhorn, D.H., 1978, Progression and regression of femoral ath-
    rosclerosis in man, Atheroscler. Rev., 3: 169.
Blankenhorn, D.H., 1980, Estimated rates of progression and regres-
    sion of human femoral and coronary atherosclerosis in 45-year-
    old men, in: "Atherosclerosis V,". A.M. Gotto, L.C. Smith and
    B. Allen, eds., Springer Verlag, New York Heidelberg Berlin.
Bond, M.G., Adams, M.R. and Bullock, B.C., 1981, Complicating factors
    in evaluating coronary artery atherosclerosis, Artery, 9: 21.
Buck, R.C., 1979a, Contact guidance in the sub-endothelial space.
    Repair of rat aorta in vitro, Exp. Mol. Path., 31: 275.
Buck, R.C., 1979b, The longitudinal orientation of structures in the
    sub-endothelial space of rat aorta, Am. J. Anat., 156: 1.
Buchwald, H., More, R.B., Bertish, J. and Varco, R.L., 1972, Effect
    of ileal by-pass on cholesterol levels, atherosclerosis and
    growth in the infant rabbits, Ann. Surg., 173: 311.
Buchwald, H., More, R.B. and Varco, R.L., 1974, Surgical treatment
    of hyperlipidemia, Circulation, 49/50 (Suppl. I).
Chakravarti, R.N., Sasi Kumar, B., Nair, C.R. and Kumar, M., 1977,
    Reversibility of cholesterol-adrenaline-induced atherosclero-
    sis in Rhesus monkeys: evaluation of safflower oil and low-
    fat low-calorie diet, Atherosclerosis, 28: 405.
Christensen, B.C., Chemnitz, J., Tkocz, J. and Kim, C.M., 1979a, Re-
    pair in arterial tissue. I Endothelial regrowth. Subendothe-
    lial tissue changes and permeability in the healing rabbit
    thoracic aorta, Acta Path. Microbiol. Scand. Sect. A, 87: 265.
Christensen, B.C., Chemnitz, J., Tkocz, J. and Kim, C.M., 1979b, Re-
    pair in arterial tissue. II Connective tissue changes follow-
    ing an embolectomy catheter lesion. The importance of the en-
    dothelial cells to repair and regeneration, Acta Path. Micro-
    biol. Scand. Sect. A, 87: 275.
Clarkson, T.B., Bond, M.G., Bullock, B.C. and Marzetta, C.A., 1981,
    Study of atherosclerosis regression in Macaca Mulatta. IV.
    Changes in coronary arteries from animals with atherosclero-
    sis induced for 19 months and then regressed for 24 or 48
    months at plasma cholesterol concentrations of 300 or 200 mg/
    dl. Exp. Molec. Path., 34: 345.

Clarkson, T.B., Bond, M.G., Marzetta, C.A. and Bullock, B.C., 1980, Approaches to the study of atherosclerosis regression in Rhesus monkeys: interpretation of morphometric measurements of coronary arteries, in: "Atherosclerosis V," A.M. Gotto, L.C. Smith and B. Allen, eds., Springer Verlag, New York Heidelberg Berlin.

Clarkson, T.B., Lehner, N.D.M., Wagner, W.D., StClair, R.W., Bond, M.G. and Bullock, B.C., 1979, A study of atherosclerosis regression in Macaca Mulatta. I. Design of experiment and lesion induction, Exp. Molec. Path., 30: 360.

Clarkson, T.B., Prichard, R.W., Bullock, B.C., StClair, R.W., Lehner, N.D.M., Jones, D.C., Wagner, W.D. and Rudel, L.L., 1976, Pathogenesis of atherosclerosis; some advances from using animal models, Exp. Molec. Path., 24: 264.

Constantinides, P., Booth, J. and Carlson, G., 1960, Production of advanced cholesterol atherosclerosis in rabbit, Arch. Pathol., 70: 712.

Davies, P.F. and Ross, R., 1978, Mediation of pinocytosis in cultured arterial smooth muscle and endothelial cell by platelet-derived growth factor, J. Cell Biol., 79: 663.

Davies, P.F., Seldom, S.C. and Schwartz, S.M., 1980, Enhanced rates of fluid pinocytosis during exponential growth and monolayer regeneration by cultured arterial endothelial cells, J. Cell. Physiol., 102:119.

Daoud, A.S., Jarmolych, J., Augustyn, J.M. and Fritz, K.E., 1980, Regression of advanced atherosclerotic lesions in swine, in: "Atherosclerosis V," A.M. Gotto, L.C. Smith and B. Allen, eds., Springer Verlag, New York Heidelberg Berlin.

De Palma, R.G., Insull, W., Bellon, E.M., Roth, W.T. and Robinson, A.W., 1972, Animal models for the study of progression and regression of atherosclerosis, Surgery, 72: 268.

Gerrity, R.G. and Naito, H.K., 1980, Ultrastructural identification of monocyte-derived foam cells in fatty streak lesions, Artery, 8:208.

Gimbrone, A.M., 1980, Endothelial dysfunction and the pathogenesis of atherosclerosis, in:"Atherosclerosis V," A.M. Gotto, L.C. Smith and B. Allen, eds., Springer Verlag, New York Heidelberg Berlin.

Jacobsson, L. and Lundholm, L., 1981, Experimental atherosclerosis in hypercholesterolemic mini-pigs; regression of cholesterol ester accumulation in aorta and coronary arteries after treatment with clofibrate, B-pyridylcarbinol or a normolipidemic diet, Atherosclerosis, (in press).

Jones, R., Vesselinovitch, D. and Wissler, R.W., 1973, Ultrastructural changes in aortas of Rhesus monkeys during reversal of atherosclerotic lesions, Amer. J. Path., 70: 88.

Joris, I., Stetz, E. and Majno, G., 1979, Lymphocytes and monocytes in the aortic intima. An electron microscopic study in the rat, Atherosclerosis, 34: 221.

Jurukova, Z., 1980, Degradation of collagen fibers by intimal smooth muscle cells in remodeling atherosclerotic lesions, Artery, 8: 275.

Lee, K.T., Daoud, A.S. and Kwak, Y.S., 1977, Methods to accelerate regression, in: "Atherosclerosis IV," G. Schettler, Y. Gotto, Y. Hata and G. Klose, eds., Springer Verlag, New York Berlin.

Malinow, M.R., 1981, Dietary and pharmacologic control of athero- sclerosis regression in Cynomolgus macaques (Macaca fascicu- laris), Artery, 9: 12.

Malinow, M.R., McLaughlin, P., McNulty, W.P., Naito, H.K. and Lewis, L.A., 1978a, Treatment of established atherosclerosis during cholesterol feeding in monkeys, Atherosclerosis, 31: 185.

Malinow, M.R., McLaughlin, P., Naito, H.K., Lewis, L.A. and McNul- ty, W.P., 1978b, Effect of alfalfa meal on shrinkage (regres- sion) of atherosclerotic plaques during cholesterol feeding in monkeys, Atherosclerosis, 30: 27.

Minick, C.R., Stemerman, M.B. and Insull, W., 1977, Effect of regen- erated endothelium on lipid accumulation in the arterial wall, Proc. Natl. Acad. Sci. USA, 74: 1742.

Olsson, A.G., Erikson, U., Helmius, G., Hemmingsson, A. and Ruhn, G., 1981, Quantifying early atherosclerosis by angiography and microdensitometry in hyperlipidaemia, Arteriosclerotic Brain Disease, European Atherosclerosis Group String Meeting, Padua May 26-27, p. 29.

Reidy, M.A. and Schawartz, S.M., 1981, Endothelial regeneration. III Time course of intimal changes after small defined inju- ry to rat aortic endothelium, Lab. Invest., 44: 301.

Sirtori, C.R., Ghiselli, G.C., Catapano, A.L., Lovati, M.R., Fra- giacomo, C., Fox, U., Majone, G. and Buchwald, H., 1981, Re- duced apoprotein-B and increased lipoprotein turnover in cho- lesterol-fed rabbits after partial ileal bypass, Surgery, 89: 243.

Stary, H.C., 1974, Cell proliferation and ultrastructural changes in regressing atherosclerotic lesions after reduction of se- rum cholesterol, in: "Atherosclerosis III," G. Schettler and A. Weizel, eds., Springer Verlag, New York Berlin.

Stary, H.C., 1977, Arterial cell injury and cell death in hypercho- lesterolemia and after reduction of high serum cholesterol levels, Progr. Biochem. Pharmacol., 13: 241.

Stary, H.C., 1979, Regression of atherosclerosis in primates, Vir- cows Arch. A, 383: 117.

Stary, H.C., 1980, The intimal macrophage in atherosclerosis, Artery, 8: 205.

Subbiah, M.T.R., Deitemeyer, D. and Yunker, R., 1981, Regional aor- tic differences in atherosclerosis susceptibility. Relation- ship to lipid concentration and prostaglandin biosynthesis, Vircows Arch. B, 36: 41.

Thompson, G., Kilpatrick, D., Oakley, C., Steiner, R. and Myant, N., 1978, Reversal of cholesterol accumulation in familial hypercholesterolemia by long-term plasma exchange, Circ. Suppl. II, 57&58.

Vesselinovitch, D., Wissler, R.W., Fisher-Dzoga, K., Hughes, R. and Dubien, L., 1974, Regression of atherosclerosis in rab- bits, Atherosclerosis, 19: 259.

Vesselinovitch, D., Wissler, R.W., Hughes, R. and Borensztajn, J., 1976, Reversal of advanced atherosclerosis in Rhesus monkeys, Atherosclerosis, 23: 155.

Vlodavsky, I., Fielding, P.E., Fielding, C.J. and Gospodarowicz, D., 1978, Role of contact inhibition in the regulation of receptor-mediated uptake of low density lipoprotein in cultured vascular endothelial cells, Proc. Natl. Acad. Sci. USA, 75: 356.

Wagner, W.D., StClair, R.W. and Clarkson, T.B., 1980a, A study of atherosclerosis regression in Macaca Mulatta. II. Chemical changes in arteries from animals with atherosclerosis induced for 19 months then regressed for 24 months at plasma cholesterol concentrations of 300 or 200 mg/dl, Exp. Mol. Pathol., 32: 182.

Wagner, W.D., StClair, R.W., Clarkson, T.B. and Connor, J.R., 1980b, A study of atherosclerosis regression in Macaca mulatta. III. Chemical changes in arteries from animals with atherosclerosis induced for 19 months and regressed for 48 months at plasma cholesterol concentrations of 300 or 200 mg/dl, Am. J. Path., 100: 633.

Weber, G., 1978, Regression of arterial lesions: facts and problems, in: "International Conference on Atherosclerosis," L.A. Carlson, R. Paoletti, C.R. Sirtori and G. Weber, eds., Raven Press, New York.

Weber, G., Fabbrini, P., Capaccioli, E. and Resi, L., 1975, Repair of early cholesterol-induced aortic lesions in rabbits after withdrawal from short-term atherogenic diet, Atherosclerosis, 22: 565.

Weber, G., Fabbrini, P., Papi, F., Pescatori, G.F., Resi, L., Sforza, V. and Tanganelli, P., 1981, Regression of aortic lesions in rabbits withdrawn from a hypercholesterolic diet and subjected to partial ileal by-pass: SEM and TEM observations, Exp. Mol. Pathol., 34: 244.

Weber, G., Fabbrini, P., Resi, L., Jones, R., Vesselinovitch, D. and Wissler, R.W., 1977, Regression of arteriosclerotic lesion in Rhesus monkey aortas after regression diet. Scanning and transmission electron microscope observations of the endothelium, Atherosclerosis, 26: 535.

Weber, G., Fabbrini, P., Resi, L., Sforza, V. and Tanganelli, P., 1980, "Lesioni" e "disfunzione" delle cellule endoteliali nella aterogenesi sperimentale e nell'ateroregressione, Arch. de Vecchi, 64: 175.

Wight, T.N. and Ross, R., 1975, Proteoglycans in primate arteries. I. Ultrastructural localization and distribution in the intima, J. Cell Biol., 67: 660.

Wissler, R.W., 1977, Animal models of regression, in: "Atherosclerosis IV," G. Schettler, Y. Goto, Y. Hata and G. Klose, eds., Springer Verlag, New York Berlin.

Wissler, R.W., 1978a, Progression and regression of atherosclero-
        tic lesions, in: "The thrombotic process in atherogenesis,"
        A.B. Chandler, K. Eurenius, G.C. McMillan, C.B. Nelson, C.
        J. Schwartz and S. Wessler, eds., Plenum Press, New York.
Wissler, R.W., 1978b, Current status of regression studies, Ather.
        Rev., 3: 213.
Wissler, R.W., 1980, The artery wall and the pathogenesis of pro-
        gressive atherosclerosis, in: "Atherosclerosis V," A.M. Got-
        to, L.C. Smith and B. Allen, eds., Springer Verlag, New York
        Heidelberg Berlin.
Wissler, R.W. and Vesselinovitch, D., 1974, Differences between hu-
        man and animal atherosclerosis, in: "Atherosclerosis III,"
        G. Schettler and A. Weizel, eds., Springer Verlag, New York
        Berlin.
Wissler, R.W. and Vesselinovitch, D., 1978, Evaluation of animal
        models for the study of the pathogenesis of atherosclerosis,
        Rheinisch Westfael. Akad. Wiss., 63: 13.
Wissler, R.W., Vesselinovitch, D., Borensztajn, J. and Hughes, R.,
        1975, Regression of severe atherosclerosis in cholestyramine-
        treated Rhesus monkeys with or without a low-fat, low-
        cholesterol diet, Circulation, 52 (Suppl. II): 16.
Wissler, R.W., Vesselinovitch, D., Schaffner, T.J. and Glagov, S.,
        1980, Quantitating Rhesus monkey atherosclerosis progression
        and regression with time in: "Atherosclerosis V," A.M. .Got-
        to, L.C. Smith and B. Allen, eds., Springer Verlag, New
        York Heidelberg Berlin.

HORMONAL EFFECTS ON PREVENTION OR REGRESSION OF ATHEROMA

H.A. Copeman

Department of Medicine
University of Western Australia
Royal Perth Hospital, Perth, W.A.

Associate Investigators:

J.M. Papadimitriou
Department of Pathology
University of Western Australia, Perth, W.A.

I.G. Watson
Department of Pathology
Royal Perth Hospital, Perth, W.A.

INTRODUCTION

Fertile non-smoking women have been shown to be protected from occlusive events of the medium-sized muscular arteries (Heller and Jacobs, 1976). Many investigators believe that this protection has now been explained (Miller et al.,1977; Gordon et al.,1977) by the fact that the comparatively lower serum cholesterol and higher high density lipoprotein levels of the female can exist in the presence of a higher fat turnover (Nestel, 1970, 1973; Nestel and Goldrick, 1976). However it remains to be shown why the coronary arteries should be relatively immune to the higher lipid turnover during the fertile period and whether this protection is confined to the medium-sized muscular arteries; and why oestrogen, given to men and women with coronary artery disease, causes an increased mortality (Bailar and Byar, 1970; Gow and MacGillivray, 1970). Perhaps the female sex hormones, in particular oestrogen, are responsible for inducing the removal of lipid by increased hepatic enzyme activity (Mitchell et al. 1979) or by increased macrophage activity (Nicol et al.,1965) including the formation of multinucleate giant cells in the presence of an increased lipid turnover (Nicol, 1935, and Vernon-Roberts,

1969); or perhaps oestrogen or progesterone brings about an increase
in acid esterase activity (Wolman, 1974) which lowers the lipid content of the arterial wall.

There is a further paradox. Oppenheim and Burger (1952), Spain
(1964) and Friedman et al.(1964), have espoused the antiatherogenic
property of cortisone but there is no evidence in the literature
showing that patients who have been on long-term cortisone therapy
for asthma or rheumatoid arthritis have a reduced incidence of
coronary artery occlusive events. It has been suggested (Friedman
et al.,1964) that cortisone acts on the reticulo-endothelial system,
preventing hyperplasia due to extravascular lipid, and reducing
atherogenesis in spite of increasing lipolysis and glycaemia.

A similar paradox does not exist for androgens, in spite of the
fact that males have an increased incidence and earlier onset of
occlusive events of the medium-sized muscular arteries. Since it
was shown in 1960 by Cembrano et al.that testosterone increased the
amount of collagen and elastin in the aorta of the chicken and
oestrogen reduced this, the tendency for males to produce stronger
scars has been accepted. Wolinsky (1971) confirmed these findings
using male and female rats made hypertensive by renal artery clipp-
ing.

Does progesterone reverse this process? Certainly in the oestrogen primed female at term progesterone has a relaxin-like effect
on the elastin and collagen of the symphysis pubis (White et al.
1973). However, there is no reference to its effect in experimental atherosclerosis in regard to this inadequately explained
function of progesterone.

When the fluctuating, cyclical surges of oestrogen and progesterone and the enormous increases in both hormones during pregnancy are considered, it is quite possible that these hormones may
have some effect on atherosclerosis when acting together, which
they do not have separately. Wolman (1974) had shown species differences in acid esterase activity in the endothelium and intima of
the abdominal aorta of mouse, rat, guinea pig, rabbit, chicken and
man and had suggested these may explain the relative difficulty in
inducing experimental atheroma. It therefore appeared logical,
when wishing to explain sex differences in atheroma formation, to
use acid esterase activity as a marker.

Studies on humans have failed to come to grips with these problems because of complicated disease patterns, and also because of
experimental limitations. The chicken was chosen as the best model
for experimental atheroma because:

(a)   it develops atheroma early, both spontaneously, and in response to cholesterol feeding (Dauber, 1944;   Gupta and Grewal, 1980);

(b)   it has a low acid esterase activity, somewhat similar to that found in humans (Wolman, 1974);

(c)   it is an easy-to-handle laboratory animal whose hormone status can be monitored by comb and wattle growth (Breneman, 1938);

(d)   its abdominal aorta is a medium-sized muscular artery very similar to the coronary and leg arteries of the human, and known to develop the same atheromatous lesions (Lindsay and Chaikoff, 1950; Gupta and Grewal, 1980).   Thus elastic and muscular arteries can be studied by the removal of the one blood vessel - the aorta.

It was decided to use monitored doses of oestrogen, progesterone and testosterone which were close to physiological to test whether these hormones had a significant effect on the atheroma or the acid esterase activity of the ascending, descending or abdominal aorta of chickens.   A combined oestrogen plus progesterone dose was also used to test these effects.

The aims of the experiment were:

(1)   to find the reason for the sex differences in obstructive disease of the medium-sized muscular arteries;

(2)   to explore the possibility that atherosclerosis was determined by an initial infective (Minick et al.,1979) or immunological insult (Kandutch et al.,1978) which led to secondary invasion by lipid and the well known further reaction to lipid.

Some evidence was obtained that a combination of oestrogen and progesterone altered the lipid uptake of the endothelium and intima, but there was no evidence that these hormones, separately or together, increased the acid esterase activity.

Attention was then focussed on the effects of oestrogen and cortisone on the fusion of macrophages to form multinucleate giant cells (Bayliss, O.B., 1977) in the cholesterol induced subcutaneous granuloma in the rat (Adams et al.,1971).   With the aid of Professor G.M. Besser, LH and corticosterone responses in the rat were tested so that physiological doses of hormones could be used.   Because results were inconclusive due to methodological problems of counting giant cells the same hormone doses were chosen for the mouse model using implants of melinex plastic and calculating the fusion index of the attached mononuclear phagocytes (Papadimitriou et al.,1973).

MATERIALS AND METHODS

## Chickens

White Leghorn pure strain cockerels, hatched on Day 1, commenced eating Milne's baby chick crumbles on Day 2.  On Day 3,
eight normal control (N-C) group male (M) chicks were killed by
decapitation.  Half the remaining chicks ate Milne's crumbles en-
riched with safflower-seed oil and half had this same food to which
had been added 2% cholesterol, "pure" but not stored under nitrogen.
Tap water was freely available for drinking.

Twelve treatment groups were formed and housed separately.
Although sexing at birth had been done, the chicks in each group
were further sexed at time of killing as follows:  2M at Day 29,
2M at Day 59, 6M at Day 87 and 0 to 5M and 0 to 2F at Day 115.
This ensured that at least six males could be killed on Day 87.
Since a pilot study had shown that significant atheroma developed
by about seventy days, cholesterol feeding was ceased at that time.

After the cockerels had been divided into twelve groups and
marked on Day 3, subcutaneous injections were commenced and continued twice weekly.  The following treatments were given on each
occasion to appropriate groups:  normal saline 0.5 ml (S);  peanut
oil 0.5 ml (O);  peanut oil 0.5 ml containing 0.12 mg testosterone
propionate (A);  peanut oil containing 0.00024 mg oestradiol valerate (OE);  peanut oil 0.5 ml containing 0.1 mg progesterone (P);
peanut oil 0.5 ml containing 0.00024 mg oestradiol valerate and
0.1 mg progesterone (OEP).  Doses had been derived from previous
pilot studies.  Body weight was recorded progressively and combs
and wattles were photographed to check absorption of hormone therapy.

The aortic valve and ascending aorta (AA), descending aorta (DA)
and abdominal aorta (ABA) were removed immediately after death and
prepared for sections as follows:  AA - longitudinal section in
order to show the aortic valve;  DA - transverse section;  ABA -
transverse section.  Representative pieces were taken from each
area (AA, DA, ABA) for:

(a)  buffered formol saline fixation followed by paraffin
     wax processing;
(b)  fresh tissue embedded in OCT (Ames) and quenched in
     liquid $NO_2$ for subsequent frozen sections;
(c)  fixation in 2.5% glutaraldehyde in 0.1 M cacodylate
     buffer (pH 7.4) for subsequent electron-microscopic
     evaluation (EM).

Sections from (a) were stained with haematoxylin and eosin
(H & E).  Frozen sections from (b) were stained with Oil red O (ORO).

Hexazonium p-rosaniline was used on frozen sections to demonstrate
the lysosomal enzyme carboxylic cholesteryl esterase activity at
pH 5.0, according to the method of Holt et al.(1960). This histochemical reaction was performed in the presence and absence of di-
ethyl-p-nitrophenyl phosphate (paraoxon, E600), as described by
Lake and Patrick (1970) and, for the sake of brevity, the whole
process is referred to as acid esterase (AE) staining. Sections
from (c) were examined by transmission and scanning EM techniques.

After preliminary review of some slides, a protocol was prepared and all slides were masked to prevent observer bias. Although
the expected progressive atheromatous changes were found in chickens
killed at Day 29, 59, 87 and 115 when compared with those killed on
Day 3, the experimental result is given by quantification of changes
measured at Day 87 when tissues from six cockerels were available
in every group. The endothelium and intima of the various aortic
segments (AA, DA, ABA) were assessed by one observer (HAC) by high
power (x 40) light microscopy.

Endothelium. The normal flat endothelial cells had dense, long
nuclei and eosinophilic cytoplasm, and could be easily distinguished
from two types of larger, plumper cells; those with abundant, eosinophilic foamy cytoplasm and larger, paler, more oval nuclei, and
those which were exactly similar except that the cytoplasm had a
clear appearance. These are referred to as normal, foamy eosinophilic and clear cells respectively and were estimated as a percentage of the total endothelial cell population. The linear
extent of changes from normal (along the longitudinal section of
AA or round the inner circumference of DA or ABA) was also estimated as a percentage of the artefact-free tissue available.

Intima. Three cell types of the intima were counted: those
with abundant eosinophilic only slightly foamy cytoplasm and large
oval nuclei (eosinophilic), those with abundant clear cytoplasm and
large oval nuclei (clear), and those with little cytoplasm and
round, smaller nuclei (round). Eosinophilic and clear cells were
estimated as proportions of a whole and expressed as percentages.
Round cells were assessed as "none", "few" or "many" in the tissues
on the endothelial side of the internal elastic lamina. The thickness of the intima was measured by counting the number of cells
between the endothelium and the internal elastic lamina for both
the maximum and minimum thickness areas and determining the mean.
The linear extent of the described intimal thickness was recorded
as a percentage of the tissue available for study.

Elastic lamina. This was described as intact or disintegrated.

Verhoeff Van Gieson (VVG) staining of the paraffin sections was
used to check disintegration of the elastic lamina in those groups
where disintegration occurred in some chickens, but it has not yet

been used to check all chickens at all three sites (AA, DA, ABA), in all treatment groups.

Plaque. Plaque formation was measured by estimating (a) the percentage by which the lumen of the vessel was reduced, and (b) the percentage of the longitudinal section involved (AA) or of the circumference involved (DA and ABA).

ORO stained sections were scanned to measure the correlation between cell change and likely lipid accumulation, and also to determine the presence of cholesterol crystals using polarized light. AE stained sections were scanned in an attempt to determine whether AE positivity was related to dietary or treatment or site influences.

The measurements obtained were subjected to multivariate analysis.

Rats

Male albino Wistar rats weighing approximately 200 grams were fed normal rat pellets and had tap water freely available for drinking. All rats were weighed, marked and given dorsal subcutaneous injections of 0.2 ml peanut oil (Control), 0.2 mg peanut oil containing 0.25 mg oestradiol dipropionate (Oestrogen-treated) or 0.2 ml peanut oil containing 0.16 mg triamcinolone acetonide (Triamcinolone-treated) three times each week, except that the first injection of triamcinolone was 0.2 ml peanut oil containing 1.0 mg. Doses had been worked out to be physiological rather than pharmacological by pilot studies after taking note of human therapeutic doses and allowing for body weight and age at sexual maturity, and the life spans of the species. The oestradiol dosage was shown to be effective in suppressing rat LH partially by the 10th day and completely by the 25th day (Fig. 1) and in causing a reduction in testicle weight (Fig. 2). The triamcinolone dosage suppressed rat corticosterone completely by the eighth day (Fig. 3) and caused a marked reduction in adrenal and spleen weights (Fig. 4). (These LH and corticosterone results were by courtesy of the laboratory of Professor G.M. Besser at the Department of Endocrinology at St. Bartholomew's Hospital, London, and information on the methods used may be obtained from that source).

Granulomas were raised by implanting each rat with 6 x 2 mg cholesterol (re-crystallised and kept under nitrogen) subcutaneously on Day 1 for those groups of rats killed on Days 4, 8, 10, 14 and 25, and on Day 21 for those groups of rats killed on Days 32, 42 and 53 for the oestrogen-treated rats and their controls, 2 rats making each group. Granulomas were similarly raised on the triamcinolone-treated rats and their controls, on Day 10, and all four rats were killed on Day 17.

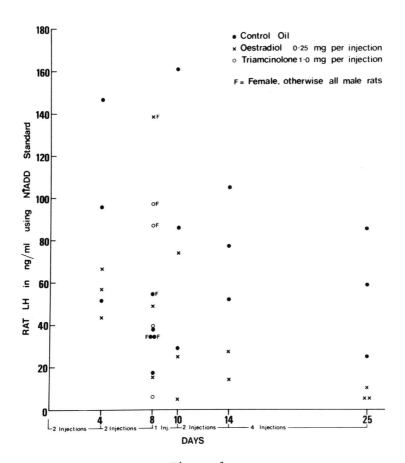

Figure 1.

Oestradiol suppressed LH production increasingly over
some twenty-five days but peanut oil and triamcinolone
had no such effect.

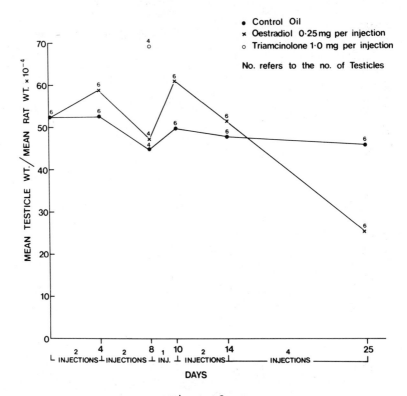

Figure 2.

Oestradiol caused a decrease in testicle weight whereas peanut oil and triamcinolone had no effect.

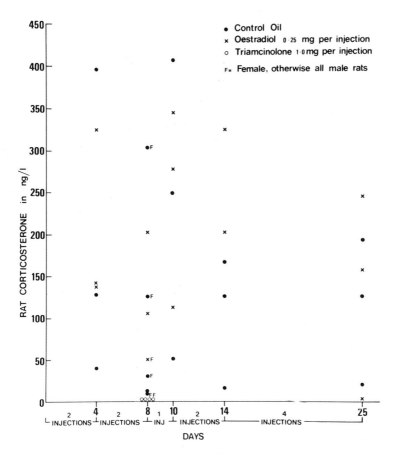

Figure 3.

Triamcinolone suppressed corticosterone production by the adrenal but oestradiol and peanut oil had no such effect.

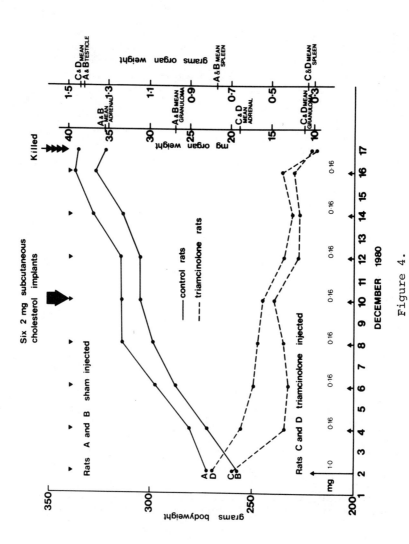

Figure 4.

Triamcinolone caused a marked reduction in body weight, mean granuloma weight and mean spleen weight, but no change in mean testicle weight when compared with sham injected controls.

All rats were killed by chloroform anaesthesia, weighed, and exsanguinated by cardiac puncture immediately.  The blood was allowed to clot and then centrifuged.  The supernatant was frozen immediately for subsequent estimation of serum LH and corticosterone.

From each rat all the granulomas remaining, the adrenals and the testes were removed and weighed.  Cryostat sections were prepared for conventional histology with H & E and ORO and selected histochemical enzyme methods, including alpha-naphthyl acetate esterase (Lake, 1971) (also referred to as AE).  The slides were masked to prevent observer bias.

The number of multinucleate giant cells seen in the total artefact-free granuloma sections with AE staining was counted using light microscopy, a grid and high power (x 40), and the total area of granuloma section was estimated using the same grid.  The number of multinucleate giant cells per unit area of granuloma was determined.

## Mice

Male Balb/C mice weighing about 25 grams were used.  Melinex discs were implanted subcutaneously into 30 animals on Day 1 by the technique described by Papadimitriou et al. (1973).  The three treatment groups of 10 received subcutaneous injections on Days 1 and 3 as follows:

Control   - 0.2 ml peanut oil
Oestrogen - 0.2 ml peanut oil containing 0.25 mg oestradiol
            valerate
Triamcinolone - 0.2 ml peanut oil containing 0.16 mg triam-
            cinolone acetonide

The animals were killed on Day 5 and the melinex discs removed for assessment of exudates by the method of Papadimitriou (1976) and the formation of multinucleate giant cells from monocytic cells by measurement of the fusion index (Papadimitriou et al, 1973). The results were analysed using chi-square.

RESULTS

## Experiments on Chickens

It is not possible to restrict the results to the hormonal influences alone because these can only be understood when diet and site interactions are also seen.  Therefore the results are described in relationship to Diet (Normal (N) or Cholesterol-added (CH)), Site (AA, DA, ABA) and Treatment (S, O, A, OE, P, OEP) and then to treatment-dietary interaction, site-dietary interaction and treatment-site interaction.

(1)   The influence of diet (N vs CH) regardless of site (AA, DA,
      ABA) or treatment (S, O, A, OE, P, OEP).

      CH caused a highly significant reduction (p <0.001) in the
      percentage of normal cells in the endothelium, an effect which
      was associated with an increase in large foamy eosinophilic
      cells (p <0.05) and a marked increase in large clear cells
      (p <0.001).  There was also a highly significant increase in
      round cell infiltration in all cholesterol fed birds (Fig. 5)
      but no over-all evidence of disruption of elastic laminae.
      CH also caused changes in the intima, namely an increase in
      clear cells with corresponding decrease in eosinophilic cells
      (p <0.05) and a highly significant increase in the total mass
      of the intima as judged both by the mean number of cells between
      endothelium and media (p <0.001) and the linear extent of this
      change (p <0.001) (Fig. 6).  Thus it was not surprising that
      both the percentage of lumen obstruction (p <0.001) and the
      percentage of vessel wall involved in plaque formation (p <0.001)
      should also be significantly increased by CH (Fig. 7).

(2)   The influence of treatment (S, O, A, OE, P, OEP) regardless
      of diet and site.

      OEP caused a highly significant reduction of normal cells
      (p <0.001) in the endothelium (Fig. 8).  This was associated
      with some changes in the percentage of the large foamy eos-
      inophilic cells in some of the other treatment groups.  O and
      P groups showed significantly less large foamy eosinophilic
      cells (p <0.05) than S, OE and OEP groups, while A groups
      showed significantly less (p <0.05) large foamy eosinophilic
      cells than OEP (Fig. 9).  In spite of these changes no treat-
      ment appeared to influence the number of large clear endo-
      thelial cells significantly.  Round cell infiltration of the
      endothelium and intima was significantly less in P and O than
      in OE and A (p <0.05), and less in S than in OE (p <0.05)
      (Fig. 10).  No treatment was shown to influence the integrity
      of the internal elastic laminae, the thickness of the intima
      or to be associated with the degree of plaque formation.

(3)   The influence of site (AA, DA, ABA) regardless of diet and
      treatment.

      There were significantly more (p <0.001) large clear cells
      and significantly less (p <0.01) large foamy eosinophilic cells
      in the endothelium of ABA than in AA and DA (Fig. 11).  No
      site differences were noted in round cell infiltration or in
      the integrity of the elastic lamina.  In the intima there was
      a significant increase (p <0.05) (Fig. 12) in the mean number
      of cells between the endothelium and the media in ABA but no

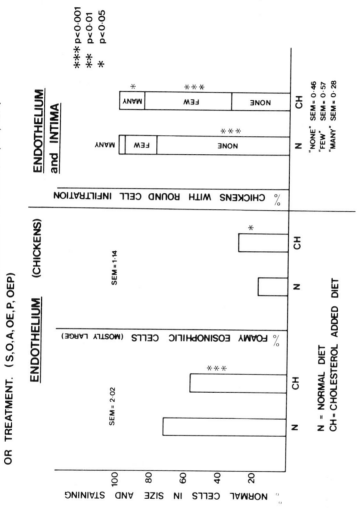

Figure 5.

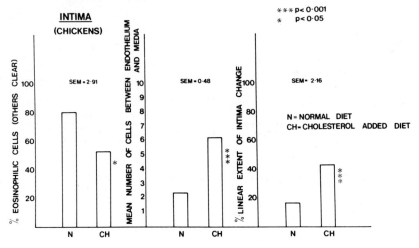

Figure 6.

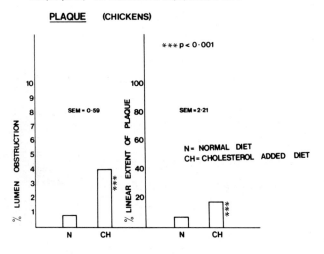

Figure 7.

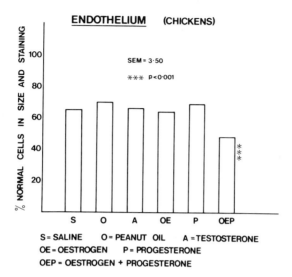

Figure 8.

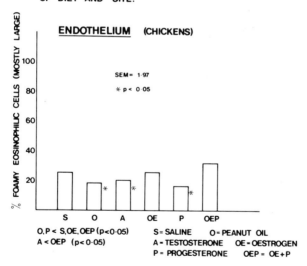

Figure 9.

INFLUENCE   OF  TREATMENT (S,O,A,OE, P,OEP)
REGARDLESS  OF  DIET  AND  SITE.

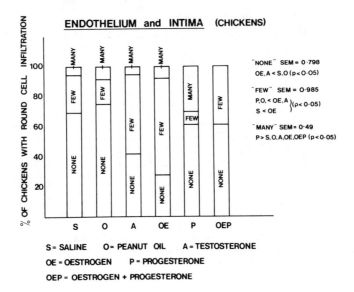

Figure 10.

INFLUENCE OF  SITE  (AA, DA,ABA) REGARDLESS
OF  DIET  AND  TREATMENT.

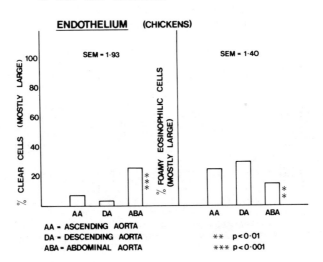

Figure 11.

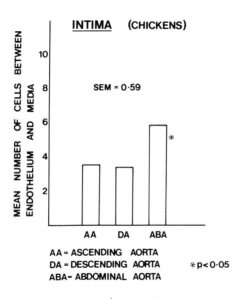

Figure 12.

significant difference in the proportion of eosinophilic to
clear cells.  Not unexpectedly therefore the most significant
finding was the increase in percentage of lumen obstruction
(p <0.001) and in the linear extent of this plaque formation
(p <0.001) in the ABA compared with both AA and DA (Fig. 13).

(4)   The influence of treatment-dietary interaction.

There was a reduction in the number of normal endothelial cells,
as judged by both size and staining quality, in all treatment
groups when cholesterol was added to the diet but this reached
statistical significance (p <0.05) only in the S, A and P
groups (Fig. 14).  Treatment did not interact with diet to
cause changes in the number of large foamy eosinophilic or
clear endothelial cells, the infiltration of round cells, the
integrity of the internal elastic laminae, the cellular composition of the intima or the amount of plaque formation.

(5)   The influence of site-dietary interaction.

There was a significant reduction in the number of normal endothelial cells, as judged by both size and staining quality, in
both the AA (p <0.01) and DA (p <0.001) groups when cholesterol
was added to the diet and a corresponding increase in large foamy
eosinophilic endothelial cells in AA (p <0.01) and DA (p <0.001)
(Fig. 15).  There was no change in clear endothelial cells due
to this site-dietary interaction.  No changes were observed in
the amount of round-cell infiltration or the integrity of the
internal elastic laminae.  However, there was significant
(p <0.001) reduction in eosinophilic cells and a corresponding
increase in clear cells in the intima of both AA and DA but
not of ABA (Fig. 16).  In spite of this the only significant
(p <0.05) change in the extent of plaque due to this site-
dietary interaction was in the ABA groups where there was
greater lumen obstruction (Fig. 17).

(6)   The influence of treatment-site interaction.

A significant incidence of disruption of the internal elastic
laminae was observed only in the P groups in the AA (p <0.001)
(Fig. 18).  No other evidence for treatment-site interaction
was observed.

ORO staining of all these sections revealed some small lipid
globules in the plumper endothelial cells with larger nuclei and
these cells appeared, on serial sections, to be those which were
eosinophilic and somewhat foamy when seen in the H & E stained
sections.  However, it was not always possible to be absolutely
certain whether some cells containing lipid globules were endothelial or subendothelial.  The clear endothelial cells when

INFLUENCE OF SITE (AA, DA, ABA) REGARDLESS OF
DIET AND TREATMENT.

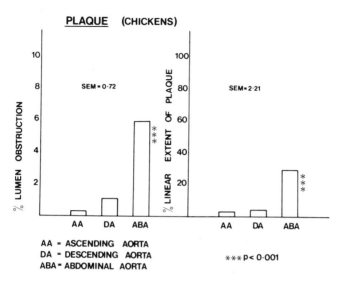

Figure 13.

INFLUENCE OF TREATMENT – DIETARY INTERACTION

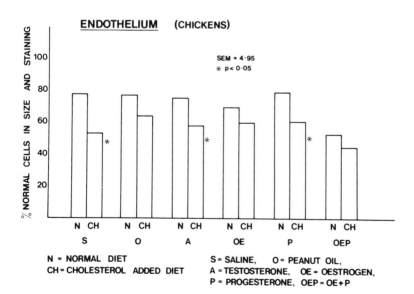

Figure 14.

INFLUENCE OF SITE - DIETARY INTERACTION

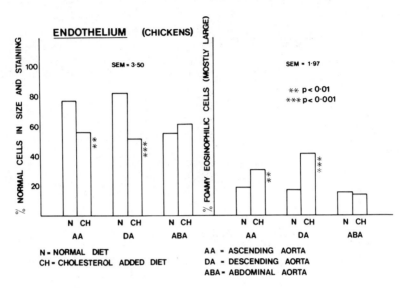

Figure 15.

INFLUENCE OF SITE - DIETARY INTERACTION

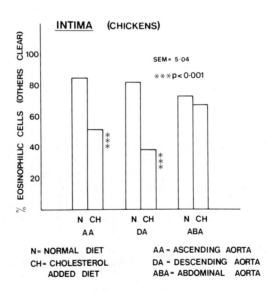

Figure 16.

INFLUENCE OF SITE – DIETARY INTERACTION

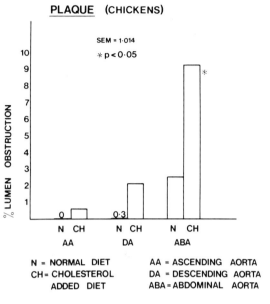

Figure 17.

INFLUENCE OF TREATMENT – SITE INTERACTION

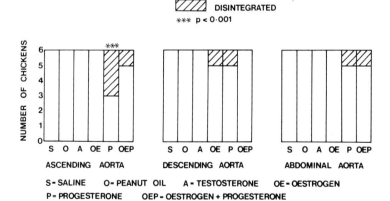

Figure 18.

studied on serial sections appeared to be those which had larger fat
droplets on ORO staining.

By contrast, ORO staining of the intima showed that there were
two types of cells with large oval nuclei, those containing numerous
small lipid globules scattered in a faint bluish cytoplasm and those
containing large drops of lipid in clear cytoplasm.  Serial sections
showed that the former cells were eosinophilic and the latter clear
when stained with H & E.

The round cells seen throughout the endothelium and the media
contained both small and slightly larger lipid globules in their
scanty cytoplasm when stained with ORO.

Electron microscopic techniques confirmed the presence of lipidic
globules in myointimal cells and mononuclear phagocytes.

Although chickens fed a cholesterol-enriched diet showed quantitative changes in cell type and cell number when compared with
chickens fed a normal diet, the latter birds were by no means free
from atheroma.  In fact, there was no qualitative differentiation
between the CH and N groups as judged by the presence of lipid on
ORO staining and also no correlation between AE activity and cholesterol feeding at any of the three sites, AA, DA and ABA.  However
there was a significant relationship (p <0.05) between the presence
of plaques in ABA and AE positive staining (Fig. 19).

Experiment on Rats

The oestrogen-treated rats at first gained weight and then lost
weight relative to the control rats and at autopsy their testicles
were significantly smaller by size and weight (Fig. 2).  The triamcinolone-treated rats lost significant weight and at autopsy had
normal testicles by size and weight but grossly reduced adrenals
(Fig. 4).  Rat LH and corticosterone levels done to check the effectiveness of doses of hormones have already been mentioned under
"Materials and Methods" (Figs. 1 and 3).

The AE stained granulomas were not easy to assess accurately
for multinucleate giant cell numbers in response to treatment given
(Copeman et al.,1980) but Figure 20 is included to demonstrate the
importance of monitoring hormone effects.  The break in the graph
is due to the fact that the experiment was concluded in 1980 after
it was known that the LH would be completely suppressed at 25 days
on the dose of oestradiol being used.  The result was interpreted
as follows:  in the first 4 to 7 days the effect of oestrogen on
intact male rats is predominantly due to a balance between the exo-
genous oestrogen and the endogenous testosterone.  However the
oestradiol then begins to suppress LH and hence endogenous testosterone.  Thus only after about 20 days can the effect of the exo-

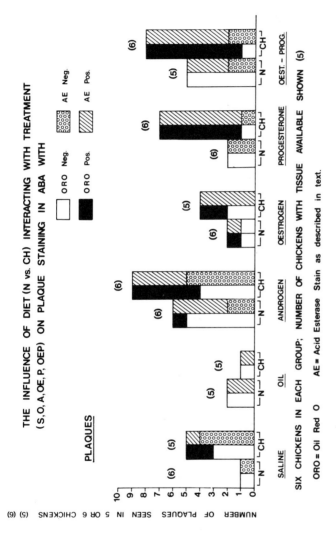

Figure 19.

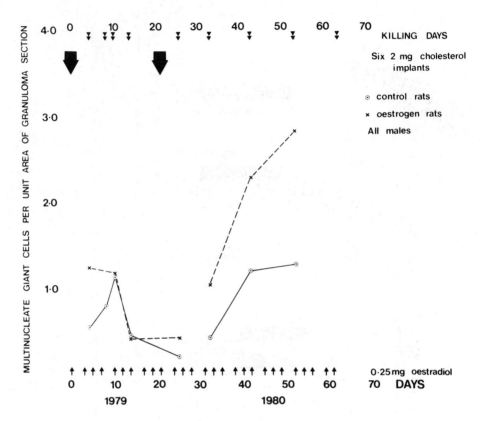

Figure 20.

This graph suggests that oestradiol, during the first four days of treatment, causes an increased number of multinucleate giant cells; but after eight days the endogenous testosterone of the rat is able to neutralize this effect. However, by twenty-five days the oestradiol has suppressed LH production, and hence also testosterone production, and is able to re-assert its direct influence and cause an increase in multi-nucleate giant cells. See Table 2 for the results of a more precise experiment using Balb/C mice, and the text of page 28 for an explanation of the break in the graph.

genous oestradiol, without competition from endogenous testosterone, be seen.

The results for the triamcinolone-treated rats were similarly inconclusive. There were approximately the same number of multi-nucleate giant cells per unit area (0.49 as against 0.56) for the controls but a higher mean number 1.46 for the triamcinolone-treated rats. This was at variance with the published results of Papadimitriou and Sforcina (1975) using mice (Papadimitriou et al.,1973) and different doses of different steroids.

## Experiment on Mice

These results are given in the following two tables (1 and 2).

### Table 1

Intensity of leucocyte exudation measured by area of melinex disc covered by cells.

| Treatment Group | Mean | S.D. |
|---|---|---|
| Control mice | 50.04 | ± 15.1 |
| Oestrogen-treated mice | 71.58 | ± 20.4 |
| Triamcinolone-treated mice | 22.10 | ± 7.9 |

Conclusion: Oestrogen increases leucocytic exudation
$p < 0.025$
Triamcinolone suppresses leucocytic exudation
$p < 0.0005$

### Table 2

Fusion index of mononuclear cells on implanted melinex discs = $\dfrac{\text{Number of nuclei within syncytia}}{\text{Total number of nuclei}}$ x 100

| Treatment Group | Mean | S.D. |
|---|---|---|
| Control mice | 13.11 | ± 5.0 |
| Oestrogen-treated mice | 28.34 | ± 5.4 |
| Triamcinolone-treated mice | 7.69 | ± 3.8 |

Conclusion: Oestrogen encourages monocytic fusion
$p < 0.0005$
Triamcinolone reduces monocytic fusion
$p < 0.01$

DISCUSSION

There is no doubt that both spontaneous and cholesterol-induced atherosclerosis occurred in the chickens, especially in the medium-sized muscular vessel (ABA) where it reduced the lumen significantly (Figs. 7 & 13).  Cholesterol-fed birds showed a much greater degree of vascular disease than those fed a normal diet (Figs. 5 & 10).

The significant reduction in the number of normal endothelial cells in the OEP group (Fig. 8) suggests that oestrogen plus progesterone has an influence on the reaction of endothelial cells which is not necessarily due to the influence of cholesterol-feeding and which occurs at all three sites.  Of the remaining cells, large foamy eosinophilic cells may represent injured endothelial cells, and large clear cells appear to attain such an appearance because of fat storage.  The endothelium thus appears to react in a way which is very similar to that described by Krotkiewski and Bjorntorp (1976), who showed that progesterone stimulates insulin release and so enlarges adipocytes to the stage where oestrogen (Krotkiewski, 1976) is able to cause much enhanced fat storage.

In keeping with these findings is the fact that the A group (and O group which had normal endogenous androgens) showed significantly less large foamy eosinophilic endothelial cells than the OEP group (Fig. 9).  That the P groups behaved in the same way suggests that the anti-androgen properties of progesterone are indeed very weak (White et al., 1973).  Thus the general concept (Nestel, 1970 and 1973;  Nestel and Goldrick, 1976) that the higher lipid turnover in the female also occurs in the arterial wall, is only partly supported, and the data do not give final proof by showing an unequivocal increase in clear cells in response to OE or OEP.  This may well be due to an insufficient treatment time but is more likely to be due to some factor removing the stored lipid at an enhanced rate in the OE and OEP groups.  There was no evidence that there was a change in AE positive staining due either to cholesterol-feeding as described by Gaton et al. (1975) or to any hormone treatment at any site.

The fact that the A (added testosterone), S (normal cockerels with endogenous testosterone) and P (added progesterone with weak anti-androgen properties in the presence of normal endogenous testosterone) groups (Fig. 14) should have shown an interaction with cholesterol feeding in reducing the number of normal endothelial cells is certainly in keeping with the known facts about the sex incidence of atheroma in most species and suggests that cholesterol feeding may be more important in males than in females in the aetiology of atherosclerosis.

Thus it is imperative to design an experiment to find out what may be the action of oestrogen (which is the main hormone in

the recurring menstrual cycles of the fertile female) in preventing
the development of disease in the presence of so much lipid stored
in cells under the influence of OEP.

Before discussing the further experiment it is necessary to
allude briefly to two further findings.

Firstly, there was a significant treatment-site interaction.
Incidences of disruption of the internal elastic laminae were seen
only in those groups with P, OE and OEP treatment and significantly
(p <0.001) only in the P group at the AA site (Fig. 18). It is
tempting to suggest that it has been shown that progesterone exerts
a relaxin-like effect on the elastin and collagen (White et al.
1973), so making invasion of the media more likely in those vessels
relying on elastin rather than smooth muscle for support and tone.
Although VVG staining was done to check the accuracy of those incidences of disrupted elastic laminae seen in the H & E stained
specimens, all the material has not yet been subjected to VVG
staining and scrutiny. Until this is done the finding that progesterone may cause disruption of the elastic lamina of the ascending aorta must remain only an interesting, somewhat tenuous, possibility.

Secondly, there was another influence of treatment. Round cell
infiltration of the endothelium and intima was significantly increased in the OE and A groups (Fig. 10). Thus both male and female
type treatments (but not progesterone) would appear to enhance the
inflammatory response to the invading substance (Kandutch et al.,
1978) or infective agent (Minick et al.,1979) as suggested by Nicol
et al.(1965). Whether cortisone or triamcinolone influences the
round cell infiltration associated with these invading factors will
only be known when cockerels are able to be treated over many
months with a steroid dosage yet to be devised.

Therefore the next logical step was to study the influence
that oestrogen or triamcinolone may have on the amount of AE in
macrophages, or on the rate of fusion of macrophages to form multinucleate giant cells. It was postulated that, by pooling their
acid esterase, the giant cells may be able to engulf the cholesterol
crystals, slow down the immunological response, and at the same
time put the lipid back into circulation as lipoprotein.

An attempt was made at Guy's Hospital Medical School, using
the technique of Adams et al.(1971) and the special tests available
at St. Bartholomew's Hospital Endocrinology Department (Director,
Professor G.M. Besser), to show either an increased amount of AE in
macrophages or an increased rate of fusion of macrophages into multinucleate giant cells using oestrogen-treated rats in which cholesterol granulomas had been raised subcutaneously. At the same time,

triamcinolone was used in an attempt to show that both these effects
may be reduced.  For methodological reasons no conclusive result was
obtained.  However the work gave vital information on the doses of
both oestradiol and triamcinolone which would influence the rats in
a controlled manner over a known time (see Figs. 21, 1 & 3).  Using
these doses for mice and the methods of Papadimitriou et al.(1973),
Papadimitriou and Sforcina (1975) and Papadimitriou (1976), it was
shown that oestrogen increases leucocyte exudation and encourages
monocytic fusion, and that triamcinolone suppresses leucocytic exudation and reduces monocytic fusion (Tables 1 & 2).

    Thus it is concluded that there is good evidence that oestrogen
plus progesterone increases lipid penetration of the arterial wall
but that oestrogen may enhance its removal, possibly by stimulating
multinucleate giant cell formation.  Bayliss (1977) has shown that
multinucleate giant cells engulf cholesterol crystals and Adams (1973)
has explained how the cholesterol is taken up again as plasma lipoprotein.


SUMMARY AND CONCLUSIONS

    White Leghorn cockerels, fed either normal or cholesterol en-
riched food, were injected with saline, peanut oil, testosterone,
oestradiol, progesterone, or oestradiol plus progesterone for 87
days.  The ascending aortas, descending aortas and abdominal aortas
were examined by light and electron microscopy and both qualitative
and quantitative assessments made.  The results were subjected to
multivariate analysis.

    Cholesterol feeding increased lipid storage and round cell in-
filtration in the endothelium and intima, and both the degree of
lipid storage and the amount of lumen obstruction was much greater
in the abdominal aorta than in the ascending or descending aorta.
Treatment with oestrogen plus progesterone, regardless of diet or
site of action, caused a highly significant reduction in the percentage of normal cells of the endothelium.  Those cockerels treated
with oil, androgen and progesterone showed significantly less large
foamy eosinophilic endothelial cells than those treated with oestrogen plus progesterone.  The degree of round cell infiltration
was increased by androgen and oestrogen, but not by oestrogen plus
progesterone, when compared with both saline treated and oil treated
controls.  Cholesterol feeding caused a reduced percentage of normal
endothelial cells.  This was significantly enhanced by treatment
with androgen, progesterone and saline.  The effect of cholesterol
feeding as a cause of a reduced percentage of normal, and an increased percentage of foamy eosinophilic endothelial cells, was significantly enhanced in the ascending aorta and the descending aorta
but not in the abdominal aorta.  The same site-dietary interaction

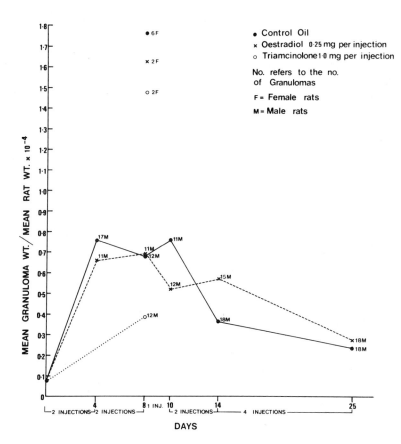

Figure 21.

This graph shows (1) that triamcinolone-treated male rats
produced much smaller granulomas than peanut-oil or oestradiol-
treated animals and (2) that oestradiol had the same effect on
the granuloma weight as it had on the body weight of male rats.
The small number of granulomas raised in female rats in a
pilot study are shown for comparison.  It was apparent that
female rats would be unpredictable models in short term
experiments unless oestrus cycles were monitored carefully.

was observed in the trend towards an excess of large clear cells over large eosinophilic cells in the intima.  In spite of this the extent of plaque likely to cause obstruction as a result of this site-dietary interaction was increased only in the abdominal aorta. An unexpected treatment-site interaction was that progesterone had an enhanced effect, causing disruption of the internal elastic lamina of the ascending aorta but not of the descending or abdominal aortas.  There was no evidence that diet or treatment increased the amount of acid esterase in the tissues, even though the chickens showed the expected species deficiency of this enzyme, but there was a significant relationship between the presence of lipid and the amount of acid esterase in the plaques of the abdominal aorta.

Male albino Wistar rats were primed with peanut oil, oestrogen and triamcinolone before subcutaneous granulomas were induced by implanting cholesterol, and then treated with these substances for longer periods.  Cryostat sections of the granulomas were prepared for conventional histology and selected histochemical enzyme methods, including alpha-naphthyl acetate esterase.

Oestrogen-treated granulomas did not show a significant change in the staining of acid esterase positive macrophages when compared with peanut oil- and triamcinolone-treated granulomas, and methodological problems prevented quantitative evaluation of macrophages and multinucleate giant cells.  However, useful information on dosages to suppress LH and corticosterone in rodents was obtained and subsequently used in the experiment with mice.

Melinex discs were implanted subcutaneously in male Balb/C mice which were then injected with peanut oil, oestrogen or triamcinolone. After five days the discs were removed for assessment of exudate and the formation of multinucleate giant cells.  The results were analysed using chi-square.

The oestrogen-treated mice showed an increased intensity of leucocyte exudation and an increased fusion of mononuclear cells to form multinucleate giant cells when compared with the control mice.  The triamcinolone-treated mice showed reduced activity in both these measured functions.

From these experiments, and a consideration of the literature cited, it is suggested that the hormonal effects on prevention and regression of atheroma may be interpreted as set out in the next few paragraphs.

There is no evidence either in the chicken, which is relatively acid esterase deficient, or in the rat which is acid esterase replete, that oestrogen stimulates this enzyme production or activity directly.  However, acid esterase is indirectly rendered more effective by a mechanism which is explained hereafter.

The cells of the endothelium and intima of arteries appear to be able to function as lipid storage cells, just as subcutaneous adipocytes do, in that they respond to oestrogen plus progesterone by increasing their lipid uptake. (Progesterone has been shown to stimulate insulin release. Insulin stimulates lipid uptake in small cells. When the cell has reached a certain stage of growth due to lipid storage it responds to oestrogen stimulation and enlarges further. (Krotkiewski, 1976; and Krotkiewski and Bjorntorp, 1976)). Thus the post-ovulatory surge of oestrogen plus progesterone in the menstrual cycle appears to facilitate lipid storage in the cells of the endothelium and intima, and it does this regardless of dietary or site influence. However, the pre-ovulatory surge of oestrogen and the high oestrogen levels of the first two trimesters of pregnancy appear to increase the rate of monocytic exudation and fusion so that acid esterase, pooled in multinucleate giant cells, can act on cholesterol crystals and other lipid material facilitating their removal as lipoprotein.

The evidence that androgen significantly reduces the tendency for normal endothelial cells to become large foamy eosinophilic cells, and that cholesterol feeding enhances this effect, is considerably weakened by the following: (a) progesterone, a weak anti-androgen, has a greater effect than testosterone; (b) the two control groups, saline and oil, both with endogenous testosterone and other androgens intact, behave in different ways when treatment alone, and treatment-enhanced-by-diet, are considered. Thus it is suggested that the problem as to whether androgen enhances endothelial cell stability, either alone or in conjunction with cholesterol feeding, is unresolved at this stage.

Round cell infiltration is increased when androgen or oestrogen is given as treatment, regardless of diet and site, but the effect is not nearly as clear cut as is the effect of cholesterol feeding regardless of site and treatment. This suggests that the round cells behave in a way typical of macrophages stimulated by hormones and responding to an immunological challenge, which could be lipid, or even a virus infection such as may cause "spontaneous" lesions in the arteries of chickens.

Once the inflammatory response to lipid (or to a "spontaneous" factor such as the herpes virus) becomes sufficient to cause fibrous tissue formation, androgen acts as an accelerating factor and oestrogen as an inhibitor. Thus fibrous scars will develop more rapidly in the male than in the fertile female and the delay in scar formation in the female vessels will allow more time for macrophages to remove the lipid.

Corticosteroids will tend to delay the fibrous tissue response to injury but will also reduce the macrophage invasion and fusion which appear to be necessary to remove the lipid. Thus stress, if sufficient to cause significant surges of cortisol, may well play a part both in the inhibition of scar formation, and in the delayed resolution of the lipid lesion.

Whether progesterone has a specific effect in disrupting the elastin of the large vessels is being further investigated. It is important to know whether the continuing long-term effect of progesterone and its synthetic analogues is likely to be associated with an increased incidence of ascending aortic aneurysm or rupture.

Finally, one non-hormonal effect which is clearly apparent in this study must be mentioned - the way in which the abdominal aorta of the chicken, being a medium-sized muscular artery, develops a different and more severely obstructive type of atheroma from that seen above the diaphragm. Thus it does appear to be a very good model in which to study coronary-type atheroma. It is different in that the lipid and acid esterase are frequently seen deep in the plaques with little or no evidence of lipid in the endothelium, perhaps suggesting that the macrophage population at that stage of plaque development, may have come from some penetrating capillaries. Such a finding is seen in the chickens on normal diet even though much less frequently than in those which have eaten the cholesterol-enriched diet.

This study suggests that the fertile non-smoking woman is specially protected from occlusive events of the medium-sized muscular arteries because cyclical oestrogen activates an effective lipid-clearing mechanism which overcomes the lipid storage effect of oestrogen plus progesterone and also prevents the active scar formation which is induced by androgen in males and postmenopausal females.

ACKNOWLEDGEMENTS

This work was supported by funds supplied by: The Royal Perth Hospital (RPH) Research Foundation, the Research Funds of the Departments of Medicine and Pathology in the University of Western Australia, and the Research Funds in the Department of Pathology at Guy's Hospital Medical School in the University of London.

Special thanks are due to: Dr. L.R. Finlay-Jones and Dr. L.R. Matz of the Department of Pathology, RPH, who provided many facilities; Mr. N.S. Stenhouse and the staff of the Raine Medical Statistics Department of the University of Western Australia; and to Professor G.M. Besser at St. Bartholomew's Hospital, London, for the rat LH and corticosterone measurements.

REFERENCES

Adams, C.W., 1973, The pathogenesis of atherosclerosis,
    J. Clin. Path., 26: Suppl. 5, 38.
Adams, C.W., Abdulla, Y.H., and Bayliss, O.B., 1971, Entry of
    esterified cholesterol into foam cells, Atherosclerosis, 13: 111
Bailar, J.C., and Byar, D., 1970, Estrogen treatment for cancer of
    the prostate - Early results with 3 doses of diethyl-stilboe-
    trol and placebo, Cancer, 26: 257.
Bayliss, O.B., 1977, Ph.D. Thesis, London University,  The
    cellular response to cholesterol crystals.
Breneman, W.R., 1938, Relative effectiveness of testosterone
    propionate and dihydroandrosterone benzoate in the chick as
    indicated by comb growth, Endocrinology, 23: 45.
Cembrano, J., Lillo, M., Val, J., and Mardones, J., 1960, Influence
    of sex differences and hormones on elastin and collagen in
    aorta of chickens, Circulat. Res., 8: 527.
Copeman, H.A., Bayliss High, O.B., and Adams, C.W.M., 1980, The
    effect of oestrogen and triamcinolone on the macrophage popul-
    ation of the cholesterol granuloma in the rat.  Paper presented
    at the VIth International Congress of Histochemistry and Cyto-
    chemistry.  Brighton, U.K., August 20-22.
Dauber, D.V., 1944, Spontaneous atheroma in chickens, Arch. Path.
    38, 46.
Friedman, M., Byers, S., and St. George, S., 1964, Cortisone and
    experimental atherosclerosis, Arch. Path., 77: 142.
Gaton, E., Bubis, J.J., and Wolman, M., 1975, Acid esterase in the
    aorta of the hyperlipidemic rat:  A histochemical study,
    Path. Europ., 10: 129.
Gordon, T., Castelli, W.P., Hjortland, M.C., Kannel, W.B., and
    Dawber, T.R., 1977, High density lipoprotein as a protective
    factor against coronary heart disease, Amer. J. Med., 62, 707.
Gow, S., and MacGillivray, I., 1970, Metabolic, hormonal and vasc-
    ular changes after synthetic oestrogen therapy in oophorect-
    omized women, Brit. Med. J., 26: 251.
Gupta, P.P., and Grewal, G.S., 1980, Spontaneous aortic athero-
    sclerosis in chicken, Indian J. Med. Res. 71: 410.
Heller, R.F., and Jacobs, N.S., 1978, Coronary heart disease in
    relation to age, sex and the menopause, Brit. Med. J., 1: 472.
Holt, S.J., Hobbiger, E.E., and Parvan, G.L.S., 1960, Preservation
    of integrity of rat tissues for cytochemical staining purposes,
    J. Biophys. & Biochem. Cytol., 7: 383.
Kandutch, A.A., Chen, H.W., Heiniger, H.J., 1978, Biological act-
    ivity of some oxygenated sterols, Science, 201 (4355): 498.
Krotkiewski, M., 1976, The effects of estrogens on regional adi-
    pose tissue cellularity in the rat, Acta physiol. scand. 96: 128.
Krotkiewski, M., and Bjorntorp, P., 1976, The effect of progester-
    one and of insulin administration on regional adipose tissue
    cellularity in the rat, Acta physiol. scand., 96: 122.

Lake, B.D., 1971, Histochemical detection of the enzyme deficiency
    in blood films in Wolman's disease, J. Clin. Path., 24: 617.
Lake, B.D., and Patrick, A.D., 1970, Wolman's disease: Deficiency
    of E600-resistant acid esterase activity with storage of lipids
    in lysosomes, J. Paediatrics, 76: 262.
Miller, N.E., Forde, O.H., Thelle, D., and Mjos, O.D., 1977, High
    density lipoprotein and coronary heart disease - A prospective
    case control study, Lancet, 1: 965.
Minick, C.R., Fabricant, C.G., Fabricant, J., and Litrenta, M.M.,
    1979, Atheroarteriosclerosis induced by infection with a
    herpes virus, Amer. J. Path., 96: 673.
Nestel, P.J., 1970, Turnover of plasma esterified cholesterol.
    Influence of dietary fat and carbohydrate and relation to
    plasma lipids and body weight, Clin. Sci., 38: 593.
Nestel, P.J., 1973, Triglyceride turnover in man, Progress in
    Biochemical Pharmacology, 8: 125.
Nestel, P.J., and Goldrick, R.B., 1976, Obesity: changes in
    lipid metabolism and the role of insulin, Clinics in Endocrin-
    ology and Metabolism, 5 (2): 313.
Nicol, T., 1935, The female reproductive system in the guinea pig:
    fat production: influence of hormones, Trans. R. Soc.
    Edinburgh, 58: 449.
Nicol, T., Vernon-Roberts, B., and Quantock, D.C., 1965, The infl-
    uence of various hormones on the reticulo-endothelial system:
    endocrine control of body defence, J. Endocrin., 33: 365.
Oppenheim, E., and Burger, M., 1952, The effect of cortisone and
    ACTH on experimental cholesterol atherosclerosis in rabbits,
    Circulation, 6: 470.
Papadimitriou, J.M., 1976, The influence of the thymus on multi-
    nucleate giant cell formation, J. Path., 118: 153.
Papadimitriou, J.M., and Sforcina, D., 1975, The effects of drugs
    on monocytic fusion in vivo, Exp. Cell Res., 91: 233.
Papadimitriou, J.M., Sforcina, D., and Papaelias, L., 1973,
    Kinetics of multinucleate giant cell formation and their
    modification by various agents in foreign body reaction,
    Amer. J. Path., 73: 349.
Spain, D.M., 1964, Effects of estrogen and hydrocortisone. Effects
    of cholesterol implants in rabbits on stock and high cholest-
    erol diets, Arch. Path., 78: 540.
Vernon-Roberts, B., 1969, The effects of steroid hormones on macro-
    phage activity, Int. Rev. Cytol., 25: 131.
White, A., Handler, P., and Smith, E.L., 1973, Principles of
    Biochemistry, McGraw-Hill, Kogakusha.
Wolinsky, H., 1971, Effects of hypertension and its reversal on the
    thoracic aorta of male and female rats. Circ. Research, 28: 622.
Wolman, M., 1974, Acid esterase as a factor in atheromatosis,
    Atherosclerosis, 20: 217.

# CONNECTIVE TISSUE METABOLISM IN DEVELOPMENT AND HEALING OF ATHEROSCLEROTIC LESIONS DURING LIFE

J. Lindner, G. Heinz, I. Mangold, K. Sames,
P. Schmiegelow and K. Grasedyck

Department of Pathology and 1st Medical Clinic
University of Hamburg
FRG

## INTRODUCTION

In this paper special results of connective tissue research in development and healing of atherosclerotic lesions during life are reported.

## MATERIALS AND METHODS

This report is based on findings on human biopsy and autopsy material as well as on experiments done on rats. The studies included histochemical and autoradiographic procedures combined with radio-biochemical assays. Details of the techniques used are reported in detail elsewhere (Lindner et al., 1967; Lindner, 1969, 1974, 1975, 1977, 1978, 1981; Grasedyck and Lindner, 1977; Schröder et al., 1981.)

## RESULTS AND DISCUSSION

In humans and animals the first arterial response to atherogenic and other stimuli and noxes can be an increase in proliferation and metabolism of arterial cells. The increased proliferation rates are determined by $^3$H-thymidine autoradiograms on human smooth muscle cells and on endothelia as well as by assays of specific DNA-activity. This has been demonstrated in human biopsy as well as experimental material (with statistical evaluations) (Kunz, Kranz and Keim, 1967; Hauss, 1970; Buddecke, 1978; Lindner, 1978; Ross, Glomset and Harker, 1978; Lindner, 1981; Schröder and co-workers, 1981).

$^3$H-Thymidin-Markierungsindex (in %) :22. Tag,1.5 und 5.5 Monate sowie
Abfall in % (vom 22. Tag zum 1.5 Mon. und vom 1.5 Mon. zum 5.5 Mon. )

| | 22.Tag | 22.Tag →1.5 Mon. | 1.5 Mon. | 1.5 Mon. →5.5 Mon. | 5.5 Mon. |
|---|---|---|---|---|---|
| Hepatocyten [+] | 3.95 | - 78.73 | 0.84 | - 63.1o | 0.31 |
| G M Z | | | | | |
| Dünndarm | 13.76 | - 97.o2 | 0.41 | - 14.63 | 0.35 |
| Dickdarm | 26.85 | - 97.o2 | 0.8o | - 2o.oo | 0.64 |
| Aorta | 11.oo | - 26.36 | 8.1o | - 37.65 | 5.o5 |
| A. pulmonalis | 13.11 | - 31.2o | 9.o2 | - 21.18 | 7.11 |
| Gelenkknorpel | | | | | |
| Knie | | | 0.58 | - 82.76 | 0.1o |
| Schulter | | | 0.66 | - 8o.3o | 0.13 |
| Rippenknorpel | | | 0.53 | - 62.26 | 0.2o |

[+] Hepatocyten : 2o. Tag = M.I. von 23 %,Abfall zum 22. Tag von 82.83 %

Fig. 1:   $^3$H-Thymidine-labelling index (in %) of various smooth
muscle cells (in comparison to cartilage cells of different localisations) during and at the end of maturation.

The $^3$H-thymidine-labelling-indices of the various connective
tissue cells in rats and mice decrease rapidly and significantly
prenatally, and slower in the postnatal period up to the end of the
growth phase as shown in Fig. 1.  These labelling indices are different for the various endothelia and smooth muscle cells.  They
are higher for the gastro-intestinal smooth muscle cells than for
the endothelia.  In contrast cartilage cells and hepatocytes show
a greater decrease of the proliferation pool up to the end of
maturation and growth than smooth muscle cells (Fig. 2).  Therefore
chondrocytes and hepatocytes react more effectively to different
injurious and necrotizing agents than smooth muscle cells.  Thus,
the first-mentioned cells react to injury from an original pri-
vileged condition, while the arterial smooth muscle cells react
"out of run", because their growth capacity and proliferation pool
are less extensive (Lindner, 1978, 1981; Schröder and co-workers,
1981).

These findings are important for diseases, grafted on aging,
and especially for the development and healing of atherosclerosis
during the several life periods of humans.  In rats the specific

| Rat | Uronic Acid/DNA | | | Hexosamine/DNA | | | $^3$H–Thymidine/DNA | | |
|------|------|------|------|------|------|------|------|------|------|
| Months | 3 | 6 | 18 | 3 | 6 | 18 | 3 | 6 | 18 |
| Aorta | 0.56 | 0.51 | 0.48 | 0.5o | 0.51 | 0.44 | 6.35 | 3.89 | 2.71 |
| Skin | 0.29 | 0.23 | 0.17 | 0.48 | 0.53 | 0.31 | 7.74 | 7.98 | 2.79 |
| Liver | 0.11 | 0.04 | 0.1o | 0.16 | 0.13 | 0.22 | 0.43 | 0.27 | 0.18 |

underlined values : $p < 0.01$, 3 ⟶ 18 months

Fig. 2: Decrease of specific DNA-activity and in part also of
uronic acid/DNA- and hexosamine/DNA-ratios of aorta (in
comparison to skin and liver) from the 3rd to the 18th month
of life of rats (details see text).

DNA-activity decreases significantly from the end of the growth-
phase until the 18th month in the aorta as well as in the skin and
liver (Lindner, 1972, 1975, 1978, 1981). This is an indication
for the turnover-decrease of arterial smooth muscle cells together
with a decline of their content of DNA in adult life, especially
in senium. As smooth muscle cells constitute over 90% of the total
of cells in the rat aorta (Lindner, 1975), the aging rat aorta is
relatively poor in DNA.

The uronic acid and hexosamine contents (related to single
cells) are also reduced in the aorta in aging (Clausen, 1962a+b;
Burger, 1965; Lindner, 1972, 1974, 1975, 1981). These results
indicating age-dependence of the division and metabolism of the
arterial smooth muscle cells in the several stages of atherosclerosis are important in the development, healing and scarring
of atherosclerotic lesions during life. The synthesis of glycosaminoglycans (abbreviated GAG) is measured routinely by the indicator method of $S^{35}$-sulfate incorporation, and declines like the
specific activity of sulfated GAG with aging.

The results of both methods are similar (Hilz, Erich and Glaubitt, 1963; Hauss, Junge-Hülsing and Gerlach, 1968; Lindner et al.,
1969; Lindner, 1972, 1974, 1975; Buddecke, 1978). So, this typical

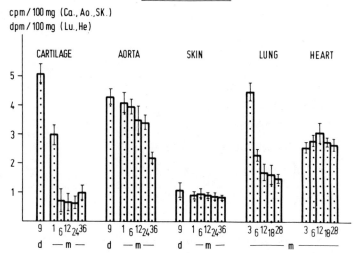

Fig. 3: Examples of $^{35}$S-sulphate incorporation rates (in vivo) as
indicators for the synthesis of sulphated glycosaminoglycans
(GAG) with respective changes of the specific activities
of sulphated GAG, relating this characteristic performance
to the DNA content of the aorta in comparison to cartilage,
skin, heart and lung of the rat in postnatal maturation
(9th day of life) until high age (36th month of life).

arterial metabolic activity declines during life in relation to the
dry-weight and the DNA-content of the tissue.  That means, that in
aging this and other performances of the arterial smooth muscle
cells decrease, e.g. activities of enzymes of GAG- and collagen-
synthesis and -degradation (Gerlach, 1963; Hilz, Erich and Glaubitt,
1963; Hauss, Junge-Hülsing and Gerlach, 1968; Grasedyck and Lindner,
1977; Buddecke, 1978; Lindner, 1978, 1981).  This fact is important
for understanding the reactions of the arterial smooth muscle cells
during life, especially, because the age-dependent performances of
several connective tissue elements are different.

Cartilage, which is composed of only one cell type, the
chondrocytes, exhibits in rats and humans a lower rate than the aorta
of GAG synthesis and $^{35}$S-sulfate incorporation calculated in relation to DNA content.  But this and other functions of cartilage,
such as the enzyme activities mentioned above increase with age of
hyaline cartilage when related to the number of chondrocytes

(Lindner, 1972, 1975). In contrast, in skin fibroblasts the various activities discussed here remain at similar levels in high age as in youth. In fibroblasts permanence of the level of these metabolic activities in aging also includes oxygen-consumption related to the cell-content (Beneke, 1971; Lindner, 1972, 1975). The same is true for the heart in contrast to the lung (until the 36th month of rat-life), as is shown in Fig. 3. These organs do not contain a uniform cell population, although both the heart and the lung are composed mainly of different kinds of mesenchymal cells (Lindner, 1975).

In chondrocytes GAG-synthesis activity is localized auto-radiographically in semithin slides after incorporation of labeled precursors - in the Golgi-field 30 min. after $^{35}$S-sulfate incorporation in vivo as can be seen in Fig. 4a. The same results are found after in vitro incorporation in human and experimental animal material. This is the so-called intracellular GAG-pool, which is demonstrated together with the peri- and intercellular GAG-pool of arterial smooth muscle cells (60 min. after $^{35}$S-sulfate-incorporation) in autoradiographs shown in Fig. 4b. The $^{35}$S-sulfate-label-ling indices can be quantified (like the $^{3}$H-proline- and the $^{3}$H-thymidine-labelling-indices). Of greater significance are, however, assays of their incorporation-rates as well as of the specific activities of sulfated GAG, of hydroxyproline as well as of DNA (Hilz, Erich and Glaubitt, 1963; Kunz, Kranz and Keim, 1967; Lindner and co-workers, 1967; Hauss, Junge-Hülsing and Gerlach, 1968; Lindner, 1969, 1974, 1975, 1977; Buddecke, 1978; Schröder and co-workers, 1981).

Edema is the first non-specific reaction of the disturbed arterial wall metabolism, following most injuries (Doerr, 1963; Adams, 1967; Lindner, 1967, 1969; Hauss, Junge-Hülsing and Gerlach, 1968; Haust, 1970; Velican, 1974; Sinapius, 1978). The immediate response answer to primary edema of the arterial wall is an increase of arterial metabolism, starting with an enhancement of the non-specific arterial performance: the $^{35}$S-sulfate-incorporation, demon-strated on the rat aorta, ½-4 hours after injection of low or high molecular weight substances (infusion solutions). At the same time an increase in oxygen-consumption as a non-specific parameter for the increased metabolic activity in primary vessel wall edema occurs. That is not a standard stress reaction because both parameters de-crease after application of corticosteroids (discussed and described in detail in unpublished experiments and shown in Fig. 5). Histo-chemically the fresh edema plaques exhibit an increased staining of GAG, as shown in well controlled histochemical staining procedures, such as the alcian blue, in Fig. 6 (Adams, 1967; Lindner, 1969, 1974; Velican, 1974; Fuchs, 1977; Lindner, 1978, 1981; Sinapius, 1978). The reason underlying the increased metabolic activities is not just degradation of macromolecules which is immediately increased by the edema, but also an increased synthesis of GAG in comparison with normal conditions (Lindner and co-workers, 1967; Lindner, 1969, 1974, 1981).

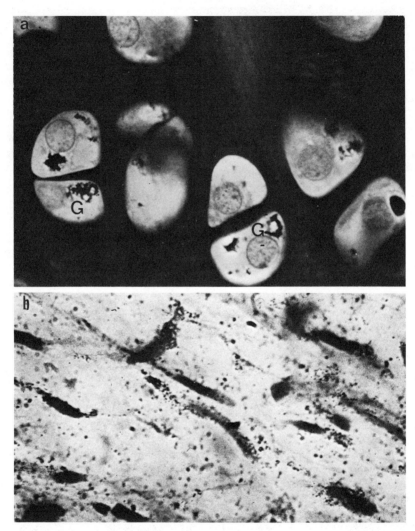

Fig. 4: $^{35}$S-sulphate autoradiograph-examples:
a) chondrocytes with distinct labelling of perinuclear Golgi-
field (G), 30 min. after incorporation of $^{35}$S-sulphate
(semithin slide, toluidine blue staining);
b) 60 min. after beginning of incorporation: smooth muscle
cells (with transition of the intracellular to the peri-
and intercellular GAG-pool)

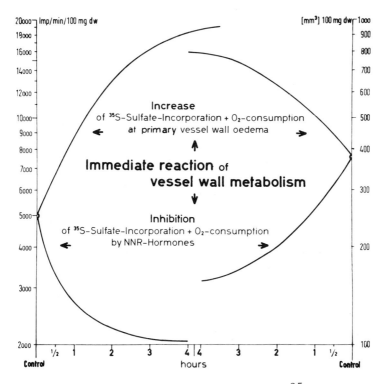

Fig. 5: Example of the unspecific increase of $^{35}$S-sulphate-incorporation rate and of oxygen consumption during the so-called immediate reaction of the vascular wall (rat-aorta) in the first 4 hours after irritation, - as well as a decrease in both metabolic parameters caused by corticosteroids.

The arterial endothelia can be lost by various non-specific injuries and then regenerate (overview: Adams, 1967; Lindner, 1969; Haust, 1970; Fuchs, 1977; Sinapius, 1978). These morphological findings can not be quantified effectively, except by special evaluation procedures on $^{3}$H-thymidine-autoradiographs in appropriate experiments (Kunz, Kranz and Keim, 1967; Hauss, 1970; Lindner, 1981; Schröder et al., 1981).

The parallelism between the $^{35}$S-sulfate-incorporation rates and oxygen-consumption can be shown during the early stages of re-action to injuries in several connective tissues. This has been demonstrated in cartilage and bone, as well as in control-skin in comparison to posttraumatic inflammation (2, 24, 48 hours and 4 days after wounding) and in rat-aorta (controls compared with findings shortly after injection of micro- or macromolecular solutions which activate the arterial connective tissue). The

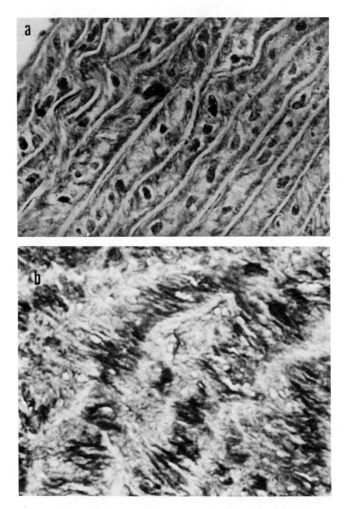

Fig. 6: Histochemical demonstration of the primary edema of
        vascular wall of the rat aorta by validated GAG-staining
        (here: alcian blue) 4 hours after irritation.

subject has been extensively discussed in relation to early experimental and human atherosclerotic reactions (Lindner et al., 1967;
Lindner, 1977, 1978, 1981).

The development and healing of atherosclerotic lesions in
humans depend on the extent and duration of the (at first experimentally demonstrated) edema which is primarily caused by an increase of the serum-protein-content of arteries due to a higher
level of permeation by atherogenic as well as by other non-specific
injuries (Doerr, 1963; Adams, 1967; Kunz, Kranz and Keim, 1967;
Lindner et al., 1967; Hauss, Junge-Hülsing and Gerlach, 1968;
Ross, Glomset and Harker, 1978; Sinapius, 1978).

The serum content, particularly of albumins is highest in
the initial edema lesions, demonstrated on the human aorta in comparison to morphologically unchanged parts of the same aorta. The
albumin content is higher in the intima than in the media of the
human aorta and higher than the globulin content at every atherosclerotic stage (as shown by the ring-test dilution method in
arterial tissue slices by Lindner et al., 1967 and summarized in
Fig. 7).

The serum-protein as well as the hexosamine content decrease
in atheromatous plaques as compared with edematous plaques. But
they are still higher than in adjacent unchanged parts of the same
arteries (human aorta of sudden death cases and A. femoralis of
amputated legs, Lindner et al., 1967; Lindner, 1969, 1981). Thus,
fresh edema plaques show the highest content of these two macromolecular substances (serum proteins and GAG) and simultaneously an
increased oxygen consumption as well as an enhanced synthesis of
GAG and to a lesser extent of collagen, measured by assays of their
specific activities as well as by the incorporation-rates using
appropriate labeled precursors, such as $^{35}$S-sulfate, $^{3}$H-proline and
others (Kunz, Kranz and Keim, 1967; Lindner et al., 1967; Lindner,
1977, 1978, 1981).

In human aortae the increased content of serum proteins
and the $^{35}$S-sulfate incorporation rates (which are used as an indicator for the assay of synthesis of sulfated GAG, because their
progression runs parallel to that of the specific activities of
sulfated GAG, Buddecke, 1978) are positively correlated. These observations may be summarized as follows: arterial metabolic functions
are highest in fresh edema lesions and significantly increased,
compared with unchanged parts of the same human aorta in the investigated higher age-groups (until the 9th decade), are more pronounced in the intima than in the media (in vitro-incubation and
incorporation with the proven indicator of GAG-synthesis: $^{35}$S-
sulfate). The significant differences are demonstrated in Fig. 8.
The values of $^{35}$S incorporation are always higher in the intima
than in the media in normal, in parts affected by edema and in
fibrous plaques and in atheromata of the same human aorta. A sig-

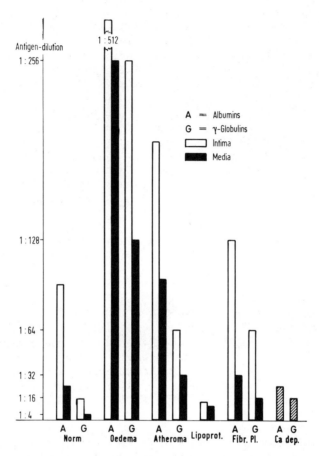

Fig. 7:  Quantitative assays of serum protein content of the intima
         and media at various stages of atherosclerosis in the
         same aorta, with highest concentrations in the fresh edema
         plaques which have the highest $^{35}$S-sulphate incorporation
         rates: positive correlation between both findings.

| AORTA | AGE (in years) | MORPHOL. unchanged | EDEMA PLAQUES | FIBROUS PLAQUES | ATHEROMA |
|---|---|---|---|---|---|
| INTIMA | 4o – 6o | 51o2 | 7998 | 388o | 2776 |
|  | 61 – 8o | 3441 | 5339 | 2449 | 1993 |
|  | 81 – 9o | 3oo1 |  | 2333 | 1776 |
| MEDIA | 4o – 6o | 2493 | 3447 | 2779 | 1882 |
|  | 61 – 8o | 1993 | 37o2 | 1424 | 899 |
|  | 81 – 9o | 1567 |  | 2oo2 | 11o1 |

Significant values : ●●) = p < o.o1 ; ●) = p < o.o5

Fig.8: $^{35}$S-sulphate incorporation rates (in vitro) of differenti-
ated atherosclerotic plaques of human aorta showing increase in fresh edema (also in high age), decrease in fibrous plaques, an even more pronounced decrease in atheromas, each in comparison to morphologically unchanged parts
of the same arterial wall. A similar decrease occurs with
aging, and is greater in the intima than in the media.

nificant decrease in $^{35}$S incorporation occurs in both layers
(intima and media) in the course of scarring of these edema plaques
as well as a further significant decrease in the resulting atheroma,
compared with edema and with unchanged parts of the same aorta. It
is clearly demonstrated that the artery reacts with these specific
metabolic changes of arterial connective tissue with the progress
of aging, during the development and in the process of scarring of
atherosclerosis. These reactive changes are much less pronounced
in older than younger age groups both in atheromata as well as in
normal parts of the aorta (intima and media) (Lindner, 1974, 1975,
1977, 1981). The $^{35}$S-sulfate-incorporation-rates and the specific
activity of sulfated glycosaminoglycans decline exponentially in
both intima and media from birth to high age in humans (Lindner,
1972, 1974), as can be seen in Fig. 9. The results from both
methods are similar in most connective tissues of humans and other
species such as rats (Buddecke, 1978; Lindner, 1978).
This age-dependency is important for both the development and healing
of atherosclerosis.

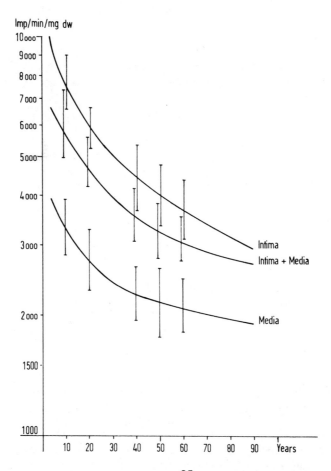

Fig. 9: Age dependent decrease of $^{35}$S-sulphate incorporation rates
         and of the specific activity of sulphated GAG of human
         aorta from birth until senium (analysis of intima, media
         and both layers together).

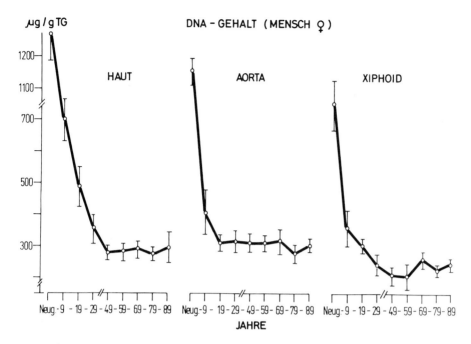

Fig. 10: DNA-content of 3 human connective tissue organs: aorta in comparison to skin and xyphoid-cartilage in maturation and aging (from newborns to senile age: with organ dependent differences). On the left skin-Abscissa indicates years, "Neug" means newborns.

Furthermore, the total DNA-content decreases in the aorta during maturation much more than in two other human organs (cartilage and skin) as shown in Fig. 10. These findings might be related to the fact that the hexosamine-content is higher than the uronic acid content in early atherosclerotic edema lesions in all age-groups, with a decrease during life (Clausen, 1962a+b; Bertelsen, 1963; Lindner, 1977, 1978, 1981). In fresh edema lesions hexos-·amine-assays measure the acid and neutral glycoproteins, some of which are derived from the serum. There again the highest levels are observed in the youngest age-group. Age-dependent increase is also demonstrated in the uronic acid and the hydroxyproline contents in unchanged parts and in early lesions, a process which continues throughout life into the higher age periods including the 8th and the 9th decades (Lindner, 1977, 1978, 1981).
Early atherosclerotic lesions show a light increase of uronic acids, but a significant decrease of the collagen content due to collagen-breakdown (Bertelsen, 1963; Velican, 1974; Lindner, 1978, 1981).

| Age (in years) | Hexosamine (mg/g dw) | | Uronic Acids (mg/g dw) | | Hydroxyproline (mg/g dw) | |
|---|---|---|---|---|---|---|
| | Norm. | E.L. | Norm. | E.L. | Norm. | E.L. |
| - 3o | 13.8 | 15.1 | 4.5 | 5.3 | 4.2 | 3.9 |
| 4o - 6o | 9.8 | 11.2 | 5.4 | 6.4 | 6.o | 4.9 |
| 61 - 7o | 7.8 | 1o.8 | 6.8 | 8.2 | 9.9 | 6.4 |
| 71 - 8o | 7.o | 7.4 | 7.o | 5.1 | 12.7 | 8.2 |

Fig. 11: Biochemical analysis of early atherosclerotic lesions (E.L.) compared with normal parts of the same aortas of humans in different age groups, increase of hexosamine-, partly also of uronic acid contents, decrease of hydroxyproline content, in fresh edema, in comparison to morphologically unchanged parts of the same arterial wall.

These data are shown in Fig. 11.

In order to study collagen breakdown steps we used the PZ-substrate collagen peptidase as indicator enzyme. We found the highest collagenolytic activity in the smooth muscle of the aorta and high levels of activity of this enzyme in the smooth muscle layer of the esophagus and of other parts of the gastro-intestinal tract compared with other connective tissues and organs, as can be seen in Fig. 12 (Lindner, 1972, 1981).

The collagenolytic activity is enhanced in atherosclerotic lesions, but decreased in fibrous lesions, while the collagen content increases in scarring and healing of atherosclerotic lesions (Fig. 13).

In regression and final healing of atheroma we found by using biochemical assays (as others) a decrease in the amount of collagen and elastin in comparison to the macroscopically and histologically fully developed and elevated atheroma (Lansing, 1959;

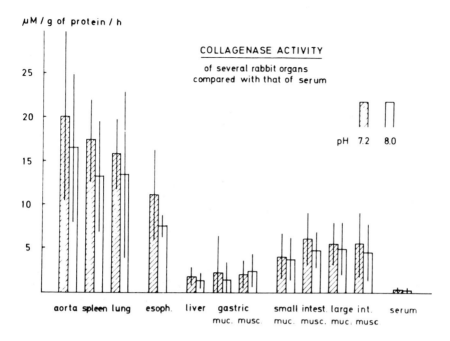

Fig. 12: PZ-collagen peptidase-activity of various organs of the rabbit: highest activity of this indicator enzyme for collagen degradation is present in the aorta and other smooth-muscle-cell-organs.

Bertelsen, 1963; Adams, 1967; Lindner and co-workers, 1967; Lindner, 1969, 1974; Velican, 1974). These findings cannot be quantified by means of histochemical staining procedures, as shown in the following examples.

The well-known metachromatic ground substance staining which is found between smooth muscle-cells and elastic fibres is typical for atherosclerosis, but is not typical for aging of arteries (Lansing, 1959; Clausen, 1962a+b; Bertelsen, 1963; Bürger, 1965; Adams, 1967; Lindner, 1969, 1972, 1974, 1975; Velican, 1974). The stained substance consists of proteoglycans with GAG, which contain uronic acids and hexosamines in an equimolar ratio.

In sections stained by Hale's or other colloidal iron procedures, the atherosclerotic ground substance stains blue and enmeshes in sheath-like patterns the elastic fibres, which are damaged and often unstainable.

Atheroma Development and Scarring

| | Hexos-amine | Uronic Acids | Hydroxy-proline | Elastin |
|---|---|---|---|---|
| Early Lesions | | | | |
| Atheroma | ↓ | ↑ | ↑ | ↑ |
| " Ulcus | ↓ | ↓ | ↓ | ↓ |
| " Calcif. | ↑ | ↑ | ↓ | ↓ |

Fig. 13: Alterations of the contents of hexosamine, uronic acids
collagen and elastin in the development and regression
of atheromas - in comparison to early lesions.

The PAS-positive macrophages can be of histiogenic or hematogenic
origin, containing and partly degrading proteoglycans, glycoproteins,
glycolipids and other lipids, as discussed by Wolman (Wolman, 1963,
1974; Adams, 1967; Kunz, Kranz and Keim, 1967; Lindner, 1969; Hauss,
1970; Haust, 1970; Lindner, 1974; Frenzel and Hort, 1975; Fuchs,
1977; Wolman and Gaton, 1977, Ross, Glomset and Harker, 1978;
Sinapius, 1978).

    The final degradation of GAG can be demonstrated histochem-
ically by the indicator-enzymes: $\beta$-glucuronidase and $\beta$-N-acetyl-
glucosaminidase, which are active in the final breakdown steps of
sulfated GAG (Zemplényi, 1968; Lindner, 1969, 1974; Buddecke, 1978).

    The smooth muscle cells are responsible for the whole metabo-
lism of GAG, collagen and elastin in arteries (Wissler, 1968;
Hauss, 1970; Haust, 1970; Lindner, 1972, 1974; Fuchs, 1977; Grasedyck and Lindner, 1977; Schröder and co-workers, 1981).

    The arterial smooth muscle cell-content decreases in
healing, fibrosis and scarring of atherosclerotic lesions.  In
the remaining myocytes the organelles active in their anabolic and

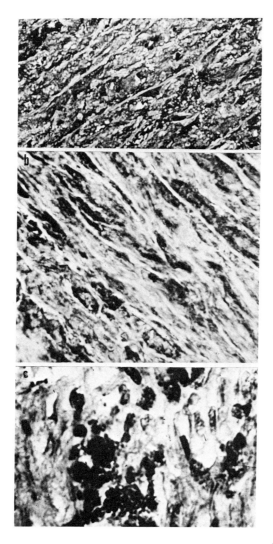

Fig.14: Increased deposition of proteoglycan/GAG-containing meta-
        chromatic ground substance (red=dark) around elastic fibres
        (with several forms of degeneration, fragmentation and de-
        gradation) in the media of atheromas in regression: a) tol-
        uidine blue, pH 3.1, b) HALE-PAS stain; c) hematogenous and
        histiogenic PAS-positive cells in the periphery of a re-
        gressive atheroma.

catabolic performances decrease. The turnover rates and half lives of the organelles of smooth muscle cells, and especially under the pathological conditions of atherosclerosis are unclear until now (Wissler, 1968; Hauss, 1970; Haust, 1970; Lindner, 1974, 1975; Fuchs, 1977; Ross, Glomset and Harker, 1978).

The so-called "ghost-bodies" are signs of disturbances in the metabolism of smooth muscle cells during the transition to necrobiosis or cell death, so that their number often decreases in these processes of healing and scarring of atherosclerotic lesions while the collagen-content increases and the elastin-content decreases (Lansing, 1959; Bürger, 1965; Lindner and co-workers, 1967; Lindner, 1975, 1978, 1981; Fuchs, 1977).

Different collagen types, which vary in their chain composition and localisation are demonstrated during the development and healing of atherosclerotic lesions. Collagen type III prevails during the prenatal synthesis as well as during regeneration and healing of atherosclerotic lesions. Type III decreases and collagen type I increases in both cases (as in arterial aging) (Fietzek and Rauterberg, 1975; Wiedemann et al., 1975; Kühn, 1977; Lindner, 1977, 1978, 1981).

Collagen types IV and V are localized mainly in basement membranes of capillaries and smaller vessels, and they are partly found under the endothelia of bigger arteries and of the aorta (Kühn, 1977; Lindner, 1981). Differences between the various collagen types are listed in Fig. 15.

These findings are important for the analysis of the development, healing and scarring of atherosclerotic lesions during life, but more investigations are to be done to elucidate the predictive value of changes in the composition of the collagen types in atherosclerosis (Lindner, 1981).

Lipids are found in the lesions because of phagocytosis and/or synthesis in local arterial hypoxia. They are stainable in smooth muscle cells of atheroma and their progressive increase results in the formation of foam cells which can develop from hematogenous monocytes/macrophages in the development and healing of atherosclerotic lesions and in thrombosis (Wolman, 1974; Adams, 1967; Wissler, 1968; Lindner, 1969; Hauss, 1970; Haust, 1970; Frenzel and Hort, 1975; Wolman and Gaton, 1977; Ross, Glomset and Harker, 1978; Sinapius, 1978).

In both these types of cells the increase in the activities of hydrolytic enzymes as well as of non-specific esterases responsible for the breakdown of the lipids is histochemically demonstrable (Wolman, 1964; Adams, 1967; Zemplényi, 1968; Lindner, 1969; Wolman and Gaton, 1977).

| COLLAGEN TYPE | MOLECULAR CHAIN COMPOSITION | FORMATION and ORGAN DISTRIBUTION |
|---|---|---|
| I | $\alpha 1\,(I)\,_2\alpha 2$ | Skin, Arteries (↑ageing), Bone, Tendon, Heart, Liver and many other Connective Tissues |
| II | $\alpha 1\,(II)\,_3$ | Hyaline Cartilage |
| III | $\alpha 1\,(III)\,_3$ | Skin, Arteries (↓ageing), Lymph nodes and many other Organs (= "Reticulin"?) :Liver |
| IV | $\alpha 1\,(IV)\,_3$ | Basement Membranes: capillary, mesenchymal, epithelial and others, f.e. Disse Space (various subtypes) |
| V | $\alpha B_2\,\alpha A$ or $(\alpha A)_3;\ (\alpha B)_3$ | Basement Membranes f.e.: Muscle, and of other Organs, insufficientlv analysed until now |

Fig. 15: Collagen types with details of their collagen chain-composition and their main localisation, esp. regarding arterial connective tissue, atherosclerosis and aging.

These hematogenous and histiogenic cells can participate in the disturbed connective tissue metabolism of the atherosclerotic arteries in the organisation of atheroma and thrombosis until they are overloaded with lipids and breakdown-products of the cellular and intercellular components (Wolman, 1964; Wissler, 1968; Haust, 1970; Lindner, 1974, 1977, 1978; Frenzel and Hort, 1975; Ross, Glomset and Harker, 1978). These observations are visualized in Figs. 16 and 17.

Smooth muscle cells migrate through the gaps of the lamina elastica interna in the intima under physiological and more extensively under pathological conditions, as seen in Fig. 18. Thus they increase the cell content of the intimal atherosclerotic lesions, plaques and atheromata (Adams, 1967; Lindner, 1969; Haust, 1970; Ross, Glomset and Harker, 1978; Lindner, 1981). Then, the hyperplasia of cells and matrix are combined. Later on (Fig. 19) we find a decrease in the hexosamine/hydroxyproline and the uronic acids/hydroxyproline quotients in the developing and complicated atheroma compared to unchanged parts of the same aorta (Lindner, 1977, 1978, 1981). But this decrease can take place also in human aorta-aging, associated with decrease of the hexosamine content and typical age-fibrosis (Lindner, 1975)

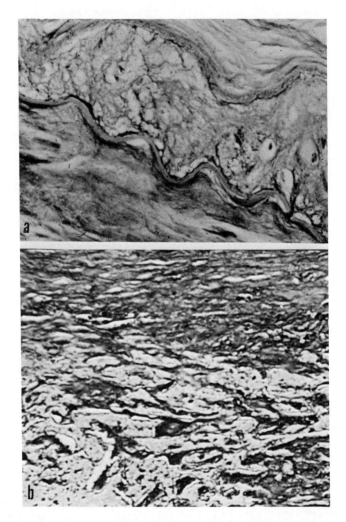

Fig. 16: Development of atheromas: a) histological examples of
atherosclerotic plaques with characteristic increase in
the amount of metachromatic ground substance (toluidine
blue pH 3.1) mainly in between the doubled lamina elastica
interna; b) organisation of an atheroma with granulation
tissue infiltrating between foam cells.

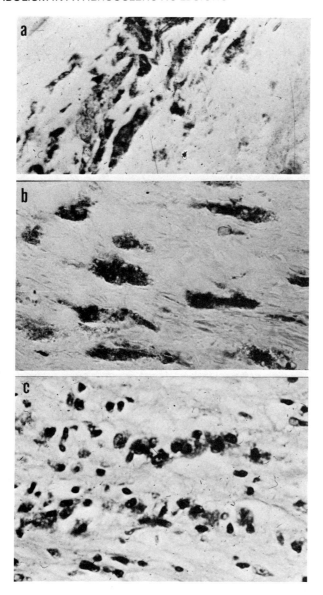

Fig. 17: a) intra- and extracellular depositions of predominantly
acid lipids (blue=dark), partly also of neutral lipids with
(red=grey) nile blue staining localized in the periphery of
an atheroma in regression; b) histochemical demonstration of
non-specific esterase in intimal cells in increased degradation of the earlier demonstrated lipids in foamy smooth
muscle cells of the intima during the transformation of
lipid rich edema to atheroma; c) demonstrable PAS-positive
ground substance components in macrophagocytic intima- and
media-cells.

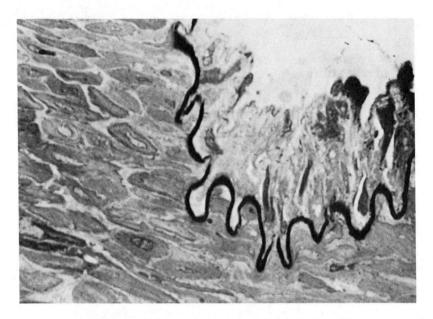

Fig. 18: Intima proliferation, partly with dark cells situated near
         gaps of the elastica interna = migrating smooth muscle cells
         from the media. Transformation of media cells (semithin
         slide, toluidine blue staining).

|  | Hex./Hypro. | Uron.Ac./Hypro. |
|---|---|---|
| Morph. unchanged | 1.52 | 1.72 |
| Early Lesions | 1.87 | 1.15 |
| Atheroma | 1.11 | 1.1o |
| Atherom. Ulcus | o.74 | 0.75 |

Fig. 19: Increase of hexosamine/hydroxyproline- and decrease of
uronic acid/hydroxyproline-quotients in early lesions
compared with morphologically unchanged parts of the same
aorta, decrease of both quotients in the developing and
complicated atheromas.

The same proves to be true for the disturbed anabolism and
catabolism of GAG and collagen in the late stages of the atherosclerotic process: the increased collagen-content in scarring-fibro-
sis in all age-stages stains red in the van Gieson-procedure, as
well as in any other scar (Fig. 20).

The indicator enzyme of collagen-synthesis, the protocol-
lagen-prolyl-hydroxylase (PPH) decreases significantly in maturation and aging in the rat aorta as shown in Fig. 21 and in human
arteries. An increase in this PPH- activity in early atherosclerotic lesions and a decrease in regression of atheromata has
also been observed (Grasedyck and Lindner, 1977; Lindner, 1978,
1981).

It is obvious, therefore, that activities of enzymes responsible for the anabolism and catabolism of GAG and collagen decrease
in aging and in regressive atherosclerotic lesions, as mentioned
before (Gerlach, 1963; Hauss, Junge-Hülsing and Gerlach, 1968;
Zemplényi, 1968; Lindner, 1969, 1972, 1974, 1975; Grasedyck and
Lindner, 1977) and shown in Fig. 22.

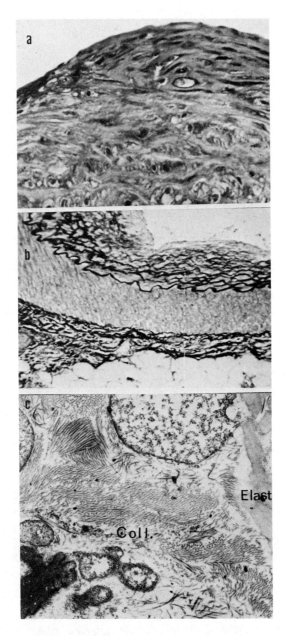

Fig. 20: a+b) Organisation and fibrosis of atheroma (v. Gieson
         stain), c) with typical electron optical picture of col-
         lagen fibres in this scarring process.

| age | body weight (g) | aorta (g) | PPH ( dpm x $10^{-3}$/ mg N ) |
|---|---|---|---|
| 5 weeks | 93.18 ± 7.44 | 0.111 ± 0.021 | 25.0 ± 6.2 |
| 4 months | 378.30 ± 17.76 | 0.254 ± 0.025 | 9.8 ± 1.3 |
| 25 months | 450.83 ± 51.05 | 0.315 ± 0.063 | 4.5 ± 0.7 |

> $p < 0.01$

> $p < 0.01$

Fig. 21: Decreasing activity of the protocollagen-proline-hydroxylase
(PPH) in the aortae of rats during the course of life.

It seems that in these processes, and especially in early
atherosclerotic lesions probably both degradation and synthetic activities occur first in GAG and somewhat later in collagen.

The increased turnover of the smooth muscle cells can be
the first sign of the atherosclerotic as well as of any other unspecific disturbance of the physiological equilibrium of the structure components in the arterial wall. The increase in degradation
precedes the increase in the synthesis of both structural macromolecules in the development, healing and scarring of atherosclerotic lesions has not been verified sufficiently until now, because
the available methods do not allow these investigations to be performed simultaneously on the same human material.

Whether this increase in the turnover of the arterial structural macromolecules occurs before the increase in the cell division and metabolism of the smooth muscle cells remains uncertain
until now. Probably both processes can take place simultaneously,
as mentioned before.

The participation of hematogenous cells in these anabolic
and catabolic processes during the development, healing and scarring of atherosclerotic lesions is possible and should be further
investigated. Synthesis, degradation, total content and turnover

| ATHEROSCLEROSIS | SYNTHESIS early  progr. | DEGRADATION early  progr. | TOTAL CONTENT early  progr. | TURNOVER early  progr. | HALF LIVE early  progr. |
|---|---|---|---|---|---|
| Hyaluron. Acid | | | | | |
| C - 4 - S | | | | | |
| Derm. Sulfate | | | | | |
| C - 6 - S | | | | | |
| Hep. Sulfate | | | | | |
| (Ker. Sulfate) | | | | | |
| Soluble<br>Collagen<br>Insoluble | | | | | |

Fig. 22: Summary of findings regarding the metabolism of glycosaminoglycans (GAG) and of collagen in early and late progressive stages of atherosclerosis.

of the arterial GAG are increased in early atherosclerotic lesions
in comparison with unchanged parts of the same vessels, and are
decreased in the later progressive stages as well as in and after
the healing and scarring phases of atherosclerotic lesions.

The synthesis-increase, which predominates in comparison to
the degradation-increase, causes first of all an increase in the
total content and at the same time a shortening of the biological
half-lives of the GAG in early lesions, in contrast to the changes
occurring in progressive stages and healing of atherosclerotic
lesions. In the soluble and insoluble collagen fractions the synthesis and degradation, i.e. the turnover as well as the total content are increased in early lesions, in contrast to progressive and
healing atherosclerotic lesions, which finally can show a relatively
and an absolutely increased content of insoluble collagen. Only the
insoluble collagen can be demonstrated morphologically.

The degradation of GAG and collagen declines differently in
the course of the process, so that in the older and healing atherosclerotic lesions, plaques and atheroma there is more collagen than
proteoglycans and GAG. So, the process results in typical fibrosis,

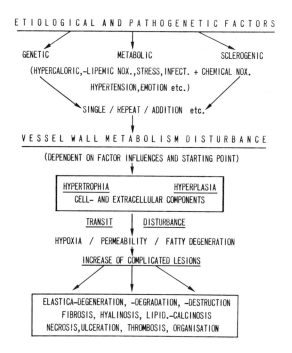

Fig. 23: Etiological and pathogenetic factors of atherosclerotic
         lesions.

as in aging with collagen-increase and simultaneous decrease of
ground substance, elastin and smooth muscle cells.

    Thus, the atherosclerotic metabolic insufficiency in the art-
erial wall results from the alterations in the smooth muscle cells
and their products

CONCLUSIONS

    In the pathogenesis of atherosclerosis, various etiological
and pathogenetic factors induce different changes in the arterial
wall metabolism dependent on their degree and duration (single,
repeated or combined).

Atherosclerosis is a connective tissue disease, which is at
first demonstrable by an increased GAG-metabolism and smooth muscle
cell turnover-rates, which are correlated - as primary processes -
to a secondary disturbed collagen-, elastin-, lipid- and coagulation-
metabolism.  In the progress of early atherosclerotic lesions there
is an increase of degradation, synthesis and turnover of GAG and
collagen as well as an enhanced proliferation of histiogenic and
hematogenous cells in the arterial walls with a resultant hypertrophy and hyperplasia of the arterial cellular and extracellular components with deranged texture.

The following permeability-disturbance is responsible for
the hypoxia, the increased permeation, as well as for the fatty degeneration and depositions of and in the cellular and extracellular
arterial components.  Similar changes in GAG metabolism are known
to occur in other connective tissues.  GAG synthesis, breakdown,
turnover rates and content are increased in damaged organs and decrease during the aging process.

In atherosclerosis the above-mentioned changes affect the cell-
population and metabolism - up to fatty degeneration and cell-necro-
sis of the arterial smooth muscle cells in both the intima and media
as well as alterations of the extracellular components of the GAG
and collagen-fraction-patterns - up to denaturation, degradation
and mineralisation.  Fresh lesions can progress or relapse.  In late
and regressive lesions the cell content as well as the anabolic and
especially the catabolic processes decrease.  There result more
fibrous scars which are poorer in ground substance and cells.  The
healing of atherosclerotic lesions can take place in each stage,
the later being more difficult.  This basic process is similar
qualitatively and quantitatively to the so-called aging-fibrosis.

The course of atherosclerosis is often complicated by the over-
lapping of progression, caused by new irritative stimuli, and healing and scarring with resulting complicated lesions.  Our concept
of the development and progression of atherosclerotic process is
schematically represented in Fig. 23.

## ACKNOWLEDGEMENT

This work was supported by the "Deutsche Forschungsgemeinschaft",
Bonn-Bad Godesberg.

## REFERENCES

Adams, C. W. M., 1967, "Vascular Histochemistry", Lloyd-Luke, London.
Beneke, G., 1971, Altersabhängige Veränderungen des Kollagens und
        der Bindegewebszellen, Altern und Entwicklung, Bd. 2. Schriften-
        reihe der Mainzer Akademie, Schattauer, Stuttgart-New York

Bertelsen, R., 1963, The role of ground substance, collagen, and elastic fibres in the genesis of atheromatosis, in: "Atherosclerosis and its origin", M. Sandler and G. H. Bourne, ed., Academic Press, New York.

Buddecke, E., 1978, Pathobiochemie, de Gruyter, Berlin-New York.

Bürger, M., 1965, Altern und Krankheit als Problem der Biomorphose, 4, Aufl. Thieme, Leipzig.

Clausen, B., 1962a, Influence of age on connective tissue. Hexosamine and hydroxyproline in human aorta, myocardium and skin, Lab. Invest., 11: 229-231.

Clausen, B., 1962b, Influence of age on connective tissue. Uronic acid and uronic acid-hydroxyproline ratio in human aorta, myocardium and skin, Lab. Invest., 11: 1340-1346.

Doerr, W., 1963, "Perfusionstheorie der Arteriosklerose", Thieme, Stuttgart.

Fietzek, P.P., and Rautenberg, J., 1975, Cyanogen bromide peptides of type III collagen: first sequence analysis demonstrates homology with type I collagen, FEBS Letters, 49: 365-368.

Frenzel, H., and Hort, W., 1975, Vergleichende experimentelle Untersuchungen uber die Thrombenorganisation in Arterien und Venen, Basic. Res. Cardiol., 70: 480-491.

Fuchs, U., 1977, Submicroscopy of the arterial vascular wall. Observations in the state of hypertension and arteriosclerosis, Experimentelle Pathologie, Suppl. 2, Fischer, Jena.

Gerlach, U., 1963, Über die Alternsabhangigkeit der Aktivitat sulfataktivierender Enzyme in Herzen, Klin. Wschr., 41: 873-875.

Grasedyck, K., and Lindner, J., 1977, Aortic protocollagen proline hydroxylase (PPH), in: "Atherosclerosis", W. Manning and D. Haust, (Eds.), Plenum Publ., New York.

Hauss, W. H., Junge-Hulsing, G., and Gerlach, U., 1968, "Die unspezifische Mesenchymreaktion", Thieme, Stuttgart.

Hauss, W. H., 1970, Die Rolle der Mesenchymzellen in der Pathogenese der Arteriosklerose, Doc. Angiologorum, II: 11-21.

Haust, M. D., 1970, Injury and repair in the pathogenesis of atherosclerotic lesions, in: "Atherosclerosis", R. J. Jones, ed., Springer, Berlin-Heidelberg-New York.

Hilz, H., Erich, C., and Glaubitt, D., 1963, Veränderungen von Zelldichte und Polysaccharidstoffwechsel im alternden Bindegewebe, Klin. Wschr., 41: 332-335.

Kuhn, K., 1977, Biochemie des Kollagens, in: "D-Penicillamin", H.-W. Kreysel, ed., Schattauer, Stuttgart-New York.

Kunz, J., Dranz, D., and Keim, O., 1967, Autoradiographische Untersuchungen zur Synthese von DNS, Kollagen und Mukopolysacchariden bei der experimentellen Proliferation der Aortenintima, Virchows Arch. path. Anat., 342: 345-352.

Lansing, A. I., 1959, "The arterial wall" Williams & Wilkins, Baltimore.

Lindner, J., Gries, G., Freytag, G., and Kind, J., 1967, Stoffwechseluntersuchungen an der atherosklerotischen Gefässwand, Verh. dtsch. Ges. Path., 51: 228-236.

Lindner, J., 1969, The histochemistry of atherosclerosis, in:
  "Atherosclerosis", F. G. Schettler and G. S. Boyd, ed.,
  Elsevier, Amsterdam.
Lindner, J., 1972, Altern des Bindegewebes, in: "Handbuch der
  Allgemeinen Pathologie, Vol. VI/4", H. W. Altmann, ed.,
  Springer, Berlin-Heidelberg-New York.
Lindner, J., 1974, Histochemie der Arterienwand, in:"Angiologie"
  2., G. Heberer, G. Rau and W. Schoop, ed., Aufl. Thieme,
  Stuttgart.
Lindner, J., 1975, Zur Alterung der Organe, Verh. dtsch. Ges. Path.,
  59: 181
Lindner, J., 1977, Glycosaminoglycans in atherosclerotic lesions,
  in: "Atherosclerosis", W. Manning and D. Haust, ed., Plenum,
  New York.
Lindner, J., 1978, Morphologische und histobiochemische Befunde am
  Bindegewebe bei arteriosklerotischen Frühveränderungen, Z. Ges.
  Inn. Med., 33: 582-594.
Lindner, J., 1981, Les modifications du métabolisme du tissu con-
  jonctif avec l'âge et sa signification pour la pathologie"(les
  "collagénoses"), in: "Maladies du tissu conjonctif. Problémes
  fondamentaux théoriques et pratiques, F. Delbarre, H. Kaiser
  and L. Robert, ed., Univ. Press, Paris-Créteil.
Ross, R., Glomset, and Harker, L., 1978, The response to injury and
  atherogenesis: The role of endothelium and smooth muscle, in:
  "Atherosclerosis review", 3rd Ed., R. Paoletti and A. M. Gotto
  Jr., ed., Raven Press, New York.
Schröder, S., Bock, P. R., Schürmann, H. W., Setiawati, J.,
  Zerbst, B., and Lindner, J., 1981, $^3$H-Thymidin-autoradiograph-
  ische Untersuchungen zur Proliferation verschiedener Populationen
  glatter Muskelzellen prä- und postnatal (und ihrer möglichen
  Beeinflussung), Arzneim.-Forsch. (Drug Res.), 31: 37-40.
Sinapius, D., 1978, Häufigkeit und Morphologie atherosklerotischer
  Frühveränderungen in verschiedenen Gefässabschnitten, Med. Welt,
  29: 1128-1131.
Velican, C., 1974, Macromolecular changes in atherosclerosis, in:
  "Handbuch der Histochemie", Vol. 8, Suppl. 2, W. Graumann and
  K. Neumann, ed., Fischer, Stuttgart.
Wiedemann, H., Chung, E., Fujii, T., Miller, E. J., and Kühn, K.,
  1975, Comparative electron-microscope studies on type III and
  type I collagens, Eur. J. Biochem., 51: 363-368.
Wissler, R. W., 1968, Arterial media cell; smooth muscle or multi-
  functional mesenchymal cells, J. Atheroscler. Res., 8: 201-213.
Wolman, M., 1964, Histochemistry of Lipids in Pathology, in:
  "Handbook of Histochemistry", Vol. V, Lipides, Part 2, Fischer,
  Stuttgart.
Wolman, M., 1974, Acid esterase as a factor in atheromatosis,
  Atherosclerosis, 20: 217-223.
Wolman, M., and Gaton, E., 1977, The role of smooth muscle cells
  and hematogenous macrophages in atheroma, J. Path., 123: 123-128.
Zemplényi, T., 1968, Enzyme histochemistry of the arterial wall as
  related to atherosclerosis, Lloyd-Luke, London.

REGRESSION OF SWINE ATHEROSCLEROSIS: SUSCEPTIBILITIES OF VARIOUS

LESION FEATURES

Assaad S. Daoud, Katherine E. Fritz and John Jarmolych

Veterans Administration Medical Center

Albany, New York

INTRODUCTION

Atherosclerosis, with its accompanying complications, is an only too common disease of man, especially in the Western World. Since it is prevalent, to some degree, in the coronary arteries of most males, even those of fairly young age, as well as those of many females, especially those over 50 years of age, any hope of successful treatment must be based, to a large degree, on the possibility that existing lesions can be made to regress under an appropriate regimen. Over the years the questions: will pre-established atherosclerotic lesions regress; and if so, which type(s) and/or stage(s) and under what circumstances? have been addressed by many investigators. Some have studied the lesions in man, while others have approached the problem by experimental procedures involving a variety of species.

The human studies have been either epidemiological, morphologic or angiographical. The epidemiology-derived data were based mostly on studies of populations which were subjected to marked deprivation of foods, especially lipids, including cholesterol, during World War II (Malmros, 1950; Strom and Jensen, 1951). These data indicated that such populations showed a decreased rate of myocardial infarction and stroke.

Morphologic studies of autopsy material have been reported since the work of Aschoff (1924), who reported a decrease in aortic atherosclerosis in Germany following the semi-starvation diet suffered following World War I. More recently, Wilens (1947) and Wanscher et al. (1951) presented data showing that wasting disease, such as cancer, is associated with less atherosclerosis.

In contrast, the angiographic approach is a relatively more recent phenomenon. Evidence that some arterial lesions may regress following a partial ilial bypass, with or without a resultant decrease in serum cholesterol level, has been reported (Buchwald et al.,1980). Also, about 35% of a group of patients with either type IV or type II hyperlipidemia showed, upon repeat angiograms, regression of lesions, concomitant with decreased serum lipid and blood pressure levels (Barndt et al., 1977).

The experimental work goes back to the study of Anitschkow (1933) who showed that plaques induced in rabbits very slowly lost much of their lipid, replacing it over a long time with newly formed fibrous tissue. Subsequent work with this species has been less than clear cut, with some investigators finding continued progression of lesions in spite of a regression diet (Constantinides, 1965; Constantinides et al., 1960), others reporting minimal change (Prior and Ziegler, 1965; McMillan et al.,1955), or demonstrable regression (Vesselinovitch et al., 1974; Bortz, 1968). Bortz (1968) suggested that the length of time of induction of the lesions, rather than severity alone, might play an important role in determination of the regression potential of the rabbit lesion.

Fowl have proven to be useful species for experimental study of regression of atherosclerosis. In the chicken, regression could be produced by dietary changes alone (Horlick and Katz, 1949) or by estrogens (Pick et al., 1952). Diet-induced lesions in White Carneau pigeons have been reported to regress following institution of a diet restricted in cholesterol (St. Clair et al., 1972).

The dog, an animal normally resistant to the hyperlipidemic effects of a high-cholesterol diet, has proven useful when the atherogenic diet is accompanied by thyroid ablation. Both Bevans et al.(1951) and DePalma et al. (1970) were able to achieve regression of lesions in this species.

The use of non-human primates, especially monkeys, has increased in recent years, with a number of investigators showing regression of at least some features of the lesions after removal of the inciting diet (Armstrong et al., 1970; Eggen et al., 1974; Vesselinovitch et al., 1976; Bond et al., 1977). Among other features, changes in lipid profiles (Armstrong and Megan, 1972; Wagner et al., 1980), cell proliferation (Stary, 1974) and the composition of the cell population (Stary, 1979) have been documented.

Overall, these studies showed that after removal of an atherogenic diet, many of the features of the atherosclerotic lesions underwent changes in the direction of normalcy - sometimes returning completely to control levels.

Our work on regression has been carried out using swine. We

have chosen the swine as our model because, with our techniques, we can develop in this animal a spectrum of types of lesions at will. The distribution, most prevalent in the abdominal aorta and coronary arteries, and the morphologic features of the lesions, including foam cells, necrosis, calcification, fibrous caps, and, occasionally, even thrombosis and hemorrhage in plaque, are similar to those of the human disease. Biochemically, the swine lesions also resemble those of man, as in their large accumulations of cholesteryl esters. Furthermore, the swine is a large enough animal to provide enough tissue for extensive biochemical and morphological studies of lesions separated from non-lesion tissue in individual animals.

In this communication, we shall present the data from our work on the regression of moderately advanced atherosclerosis in the swine abdominal aorta produced by injury and atherogenic diet, the effects of moderate diet and clofibrate on the regression of swine atherosclerosis produced by atherogenic diet without injury, the sequential morphological and biochemical changes occurring during the regression phase of the very advanced diet-injury induced atheromata, and finally, we shall present preliminary data on the possible role of macrophages and hydrolytic enzymes on the removal of necrotic debris from the atheroma.


MATERIALS AND METHODS

The protocols for lesion induction, killing of the swine and the methodology for the study of the various morphological and biochemical features of the aortic lesions have been previously reported (Daoud et al., 1976; Fritz et al., 1976; Jarmolych et al., 1978; Augustyn et al., 1978; Daoud et al., 1981; Fritz et al., 1981).

Moderately advanced atherosclerosis was produced in the abdominal aortas of miniature swine by a combination of injury, in the form of abrasion with a balloon catheter, and an atherogenic diet administered for four months. The diet in this case was semi-synthetic and included 22 g cholesterol and 11 g sodium cholate per day. At the end of the 4 months induction period, some animals were sacrificed as a reference group and the remaining swine were transferred to a hog mash diet for fourteen months and then killed. Control animals received abrasion, but were maintained on hog mash throughout the experiment. The abdominal aorta was divided longitudinally into two halves, one half for morphological studies and the other half for chemical analysis. The half for morphologic studies was stained with Sudan IV. After fixation, the entire half was cut into longitudinal segments 2.0 cm long and 2.0 mm wide. All segments were imbedded and cut. From the half destined for chemical studies the lesions were meticulously dissected from non-lesion areas and analyses were carried out on both lesion and non-

lesion tissues.  The morphologic assessment included: the total area
of the aorta grossly involved in sudanophilic lesions; histologic
characterization of the lesions; measurements of the lesion and wall
thickness and autoradiographic identification of DNA synthesizing
cells.  The biochemical features investigated in both lesion and non-
lesion areas included the concentration of various lipid classes,
DNA and collagen, and the rate of DNA and protein synthesis.

In the clofibrate study, early proliferative coronary and aortic atherosclerotic lesions were produced in swine by feeding them
the same atherogenic (HL) diet only, with no added injury.  After
17 months of the atherogenic diet, one group of animals was killed
(reference group).  The remaining animals were divided into two
groups.  One group was maintained on a dietary regimen that resulted
in a serum cholesterol level of approximately 200 mg/dl and the
other was fed the same diet with the addition of 2 g clofibrate
daily.  The latter regimen resulted in serum cholesterol levels of
approximately 100 mg/dl.  Morphological studies were carried out on
the coronary arteries while the biochemical studies were carried
out on the aorta using the same parameters as those of the experiment mentioned above.

The three major coronary arteries of each heart were resected,
opened longitudinally and stained with Sudan IV.  The proximal 5 cm
of the anterior descending and circumflex branches of the left coronary and the right coronary artery were cut at 0.5 cm intervals
and all 10 segments were studied microscopically.  As in the previous experiment, the lesions from the aorta were dissected from
the adjacent non-lesion areas and chemical analyses were performed
on both types of tissue.

In the sequential studies, a group of Yorkshire swine were
placed on a hyperlipidemic diet following denudation of the abdominal aorta with a balloon-catheter.  The diet contained 11 g cholesterol per day.  Most of the fat was in the form of lard.  Other
swine were also ballooned and placed on a mash diet to serve as
controls.  After 6 months' feeding of the respective diets, a group
of HL diet-fed swine was sacrificed as a reference group, together
with a group of mash-fed control animals.  The remaining swine were
put on mash diet and divided into 3 groups of equal numbers.  Of
these, one group was sacrificed at 6 weeks, another at 5 months
and the 3rd at 14 months.  At each time, 3 control animals were
also sacrificed.  We carried out on the abdominal aortas the same
morphological and biochemical studies as described in the first
experiment, and added to the morphologic studies semi-quantitative
appraisal of the extent of necrosis, and of the numbers of foam
cells and macrophages.  Selected areas were also studied for the
presence of non-specific esterase at the light and electron microscopic levels.  The biochemical determinations included, in addition to the features studied in the regression of the moderately

advanced lesions, the synthesis of collagen, glycosaminoglycans and
various lipid classes.

In this sequential study we also carried out extensive studies
of calcification which included light and electron microscopy, chemical determination and energy dispersive analysis.

For the morphological study of calcification, tissues were
fixed in calcium-free 10% buffered formalin (for light microscopy)
or dilute Karnovsky's fixative for electron microscopy. Calcium
deposits were studied on the light microscopic level by both hematoxylin and eosin and Von Kossa stained sections, although it is
recognized that neither of these stains is specific for calcium.
In electron microscopic studies only sections unstained with either
lead or uranyl ions were used. Further, since substances other than
calcium are electron dense, the calcium identity of a structure was
tested by its susceptibility to removal by EDTA or EGTA. Appropriate areas were photographed, the grids floated on one of the chelat-
ing solutions, rinsed, dried and rephotographed. Disappearance of
the electron-dense structure after this treatment was considered
supportive of its calcium identity. Energy dispersive analysis was
carried out on grossly visible "calcified" agglomerations in the
atherosclerotic plaques.

## Study of Hydrolytic Enzymatic Activities of Progression Lesions, Adjacent Non-Lesion and Control Non-Lesion Tissues

The activity of cholesteryl ester hydrolase was measured by a
modification of the methods of Kothari et al.(1973) and Takano et
al.(1974). Because of the large amounts of endogenous cholesteryl
ester demonstrated in the lesions in the sequential study, the enzyme from each tissue was extracted from an acetone powder in 0.5 M
phosphate buffer, pH 6.2. DNA content of the residue was determined
by the Ceriotti method, protein content of the enzyme by the Lowry
method. Duplicate 4-hr and one zero time samples were assayed using
a micellar substrate of $^{14}$C-cholesteryl oleate, sodium taurocholate
and acetate-acetic acid buffer, pH 4.25. The incubation was ter-
minated with chloroform-methanol, followed by distilled water, the
lipid phase separated and chromatographed on silica gel G, and the
free cholesterol eluted and counted in a scintillation counter.

The activity of β-glucuronidase was assayed by a modification
of the method of Goldbarg (1959). The enzyme preparation was extracted in 0.9% NaCl, pH 7.0, and aliquots were also used for determination of collagenolytic activity. Triton X-100 was added to a
final concentration of 0.1%. DNA was determined on the residue,
protein on the extract. Duplicate 3-hr samples were incubated at
50°C, with 6-Br-2 naphthyl-β-D-glucuronide in 0.1 M acetate buffer,
pH 4.5, as substrate. Controls were zero time samples. Following
incubation, color was developed with O-dianisidine, extracted with

chloroform and measured spectrophotometrically.  Values were cor-
rected for protein adsorption.

Collagenolytic activity was assayed as follows:  enzyme extracted in 0.9% NaCl was used for either pH 7.8 or pH 3.5 activity,
in the presence of the appropriate buffer, Tris-HCL with $CaCl_2$ or
acetate buffer with cysteine and EDTA, with insoluble collagen as
substrate.  Following a 24-hr incubation at $37^{\circ}C$ the supernatant
was hydrolyzed and hydroxyproline concentration determined after
correction by subtraction of the hydroxyproline content of both enzyme and substrate blanks.

All activities were expressed on a µg DNA basis.

## Study of Phagocytosis

The phagocytic activity of lesion cells was demonstrated by a
modification of the procedure of Schaffner  et al.(1980).  All glass-
ware was siliconized.  Lesions were dissected free from the adjacent
and subjacent non-lesion tissue, transferred to a drop of Hank's bal-
anced salt solution (HBSS) on a Teflon pad, and exhaustively teased
with two 23 gauge needles.  The liquid and tissue residue were then
transferred to a conical centrifuge tube, using a wide-bore pipet,
allowed to stand 2 min, and the supernatant transferred to a Leighton tube, and incubated one hour at 37 C.  The unattached cells were
removed, the cell layer washed in HBSS and a suspension of opsonized
yeast particles applied.  After 2 hrs incubation the yeast were removed, the cells washed in HBSS and stained with Wright's stain.
The number of internalized yeast was assessed microscopically.

Histochemical demonstration of non-specific esterase activity
was performed by a modification of the method of Yam  et al. (1971),
on the light microscopic level using α-naphthyl acetate or 5-bromo-
indoxyl acetate as substrates.  On the ultrastructural level, the
method used was an adaptation of the procedure of Delellis and Fishman (1965), with 5-bromoindoxyl acetate as substrate (Fritz  et al.,
1980).

## RESULTS

## Study of Moderately Advanced Atherosclerotic Lesions

At the initiation of the experiment the serum cholesterol levels of the various groups were around 70 mg/dl.  After two months
on HL diet, the levels were over 800 mg/dl.  When the swine of the
regression group were shifted to a mash diet, their serum cholesterol levels came down to values similar to those of the mash controls.

On gross examination, the aortas from the reference group animals showed focal raised lesions distributed throughout the entire abdominal aorta. These varied in size from a few millimeters to over 1.0 cm in greatest dimension and were elevated, up to 2.0 mm above the intimal surface. The mean percentage of the surface area stained with Sudan IV was 20%. The aortas from the other groups, including the regression group, were grossly similar to one another and showed, in general, a smooth intimal surface with occasional focal raised lesions and little or no sudanophilia.

On microscopic examination, the reference group revealed a spectrum ranging from normal intima to very advanced complicated lesions. Proliferative foam cell lesions were abundant, being present virtually in all sections examined. Lesions showing necrosis, with or without calcification (Fig. 1-A), hemorrhage in plaque and thrombosis were present in approximately one-fourth of the segments examined. These atheromas had large necrotic centers composed of amorphous material, cell debris and cholesterol clefts. The necrotic center was surrounded by spindle and foam cells, with a fibrous cap at the luminal aspect. Oil red O-stained frozen sections showed extensive intracellular and extracellular lipid accumulation in the necrotic center and, to a lesser degree, in the fibrous cap. The histological pictures of the two mash control groups and of the

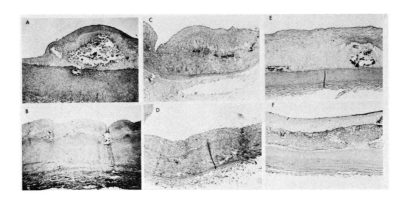

Figure 1.

In the upper panel are representative lesions from the reference groups of the moderately advanced lesion (A), the clofibrate (C) and the sequential (E) studies. In the lower panel are corresponding regression lesion (B, D & F). Note virtually complete disappearance of necrosis in all regression lesions. In the moderately advanced and clofibrate group the regressed lesions are significantly smaller. There is increased calcification in the regressed lesion from the sequential study. Hematoxylin-eosin stain.

regression group were very similar.  Varying degrees of intimal thickening (Fig. 1-B) were present.  In general, the intimal surface was flat, the cells were largely fusiform with an occasional small accumulation of foam cells at the base of the lesion.  These were more abundant in the regression than in the mash groups.  Necrosis was virtually absent.  However, calcification was common in the regression aortas although the size of the calcific foci appeared smaller than in the reference group.

Quantitative morphologic data disclosed that at the end of the regression period there was a significant decrease in the thickness of the lesion, (Table I) sudanophilia had virtually disappeared, and atheromata (necrotic lesions) were almost absent in the regression group, as were thrombosis and hemorrhage in plaque.  Cell proliferation, as judged by the number of labelled cells in autoradiographs was less pronounced in this group.  There was no decrease in the number of segments showing calcification.

Chemical studies (Table I) showed that the regressed lesions had decreased concentrations of DNA, total and esterified cholesterol and phospholipids and a lower level of DNA synthesis but no change in the concentrations of free cholesterol or triglycerides and level of protein synthesis.  Collagen concentration had increased.  In most of the anatomical and chemical features, the regressed lesions did not differ greatly from the tissues from the abdominal aortas of the animals that had received only a mash diet for 18 months after mechanical injury.

## Table I

SUMMARY OF MEAN LESION
BIOCHEMICAL OR MORPHOLOGICAL DATA

| | MODERATELY SEVERE LESION STUDY | | MODERATE DIET & CLOFIBRATE STUDY | | | SEQUENTIAL STUDY OF VERY SEVERE LESIONS | | | |
|---|---|---|---|---|---|---|---|---|---|
| | REF.[†] | REGR.[††] (14 mos) | REF.[†] | REGR.[††] NO CLO-FIBRATE (12 mos) | REGR.[††] PLUS CLO-FIBRATE (12 mos) | REF.[†] | REGR[††] (6 wks) | REGR[††] (5 mos) | REGR[††] (14 mos) |
| CHOLESTEROL CONCENTRATION ($\mu g$/mg dry wt) TOTAL | 15.0 | 3.8* | 29.5 | 37.2· | 18.3 | 107.8 | 63.5 | 53.0 | 55.8 |
| ESTERIFIED | 11.2 | 0.4* | 18.8 | 15.2 | 7.6* | 74.5 | 50.0 | 26.1* | 27.6 |
| DNA CONCENTRATION ($\mu g$/mg dry wt) | 6.6 | 4.2* | 6.4 | 3.9* | 4.0* | 3.3 | 3.6 | 2.7 | 2.4* |
| SYNTHESIS (dpm $^3$H-Thymidine / $\mu g$ DNA) | 846 | 201* | 194 | 96 | 71* | 2,302 | 3,776 | 1,108 | 290* |
| CALCIUM a) No. of calcified areas or b) $\mu g$/mg dry wt | (a) 28 | (a) 48 | (a) 36.7 | (a) 45.8 | (a) 26.6 | (b) 9.1 | (b) 55.5 | 87.2* | 128.6* |
| LESION THICKNESS / MEDIA THICKNESS | 0.65 | 0.29* | 0.42 | 0.44 | 0.24* | 1.27 | 1.27 | 0.88 | 1.22 |

†  Reference

††  Regression

*  Significantly different from reference value

Effects of Moderate Diet and Clofibrate on Swine Atherosclerosis

In the study cited above, regression of atherosclerotic lesions was accomplished by a drastic change of the diet which is not applicable to man.  In this experiment we studied the effects of 12 mos of a dietary regimen, that resulted in serum cholesterol levels similar to those of the young American males, on the fate of swine atherosclerosis produced by feeding the animals a high cholesterol diet for 17 months without balloon injury.  Further, these effects were compared with those obtained from the addition of clofibrate to the same dietary regimen.  The serum cholesterol levels of these animals in the latter regimen were similar to those of mash-fed swine.

Gross examination of the Sudan IV-stained coronary arteries showed no sudanophilia in the arteries of the mash-fed animals. Although there was some variability among the other 3 groups, arteries of animals from the reference group were significantly more sudanophilic than those of the other 2 groups.  Raised lesions were observed in all groups.  However, they were less extensive and smaller in the clofibrate group.  In fact, in the latter group, several arteries had smooth intimal surfaces.  No lesions were seen in the arteries of the mash-fed animals.

On microscopic examination, arteries from the reference group presented a spectrum ranging from normal intima to large foam cell lesions with or without calcification (Fig. 1-C).  In some instances, such lesions displayed a fibrous cap.  Occasional lesions showed small foci of necrosis, but no hemorrhage in plaque or thrombosis were noted.  Sections of arteries from animals of the moderate regression diet (without clofibrate) regimen disclosed that the lesion was more fibrotic, containing fewer foam cells.  Three of eight hearts in this group had no foam cell lesions at all.  Here, also, only a few lesions showed small foci of necrosis.  The histologic appearance of the lesions in the clofibrate-treated group showed them to be composed almost exclusively of spindle cells (Fig. 1-D). Only an occasional collection of foam cells was noted in a few lesions.  No necrosis was evident.  The histologic picture was similar to that found in the regression group of the previous experiment.

Quantitative analysis (Table I) showed that morphologically the moderate "regression" diet did not result in a decrease in the size of the lesion, but it did prevent their progression.  The addition of clofibrate therapy caused regression that involved a significant decrease in the size of the lesion, gross sudanophilia and in the amount of lipid as seen in the oil red O-stained sections.  Biochemically, the moderate diet alone prevented progression except for accumulation of free cholesterol and total protein and collagen synthesis, and caused a decrease in DNA concentration to non-lesion levels.  The addition of clofibrate therapy enhanced regression with

a significant decrease in DNA and esterified cholesterol concentration and in rate of DNA synthesis.

## Sequential Study of Atherosclerotic Lesions During Regression

The mean level of serum cholesterol of the reference group at
the time of killing was over 700 mg/dl. At two weeks after withdrawal of the HC diet, the mean level of serum cholesterol
of the regression swine was approximately 200 mg/dl and after one
month it returned approximately to control levels.

In the mash control animals, the abdominal aortas grossly and
microscopically were similar to those in the previous experiments.

Grossly, the abdominal aortas from the reference group showed
flat and raised lesions which were extensively sudanophilic when
the vessels were stained with Sudan IV. Many of the lesions were
grossly calcified. Histologically, the flat lesions were mainly
foam cell lesions. While some of the raised lesions were of the
proliferative foam cell type, most were of the atheroma type (Fig.
1-E). These contained large necrotic centers with cholesterol
clefts. The necrotic center was surrounded by spindle and foam
cells and a thin fibrous cap. A few round cells with eosinophilic
cytoplasm were also present. By electron microscopy, these round
cells disclosed many of the features of macrophages, including
microvilli, a large Golgi apparatus and lysosome-like structures.
Many of the atheroma-type lesions were heavily calcified.

Electron microscopic studies of calcified atheromata revealed
round or oval electron dense bodies, often folded or shrunken,
measuring up to several microns in diameter. They sometimes contained a central core of amorphous electron dense particles and
needle-shaped crystals the latter often associated with smaller
vesicular inclusions. There were also spherical aggregates of
granular or amorphous electron dense precipitates. Supporting the
calcium identity of these electron dense structures was the finding
that they are removed by 1 ½ hr exposure to EDTA or EGTA. Similar
structures in the aging aortic valve were described by Kim (1976)
and Kim and Trump (1975) who suggested that the calcium deposition
takes place on products of cellular degradation. In our study,
intracellular calcific bodies, similar to the extracellular structures, were commonly seen, generally in cells with some evidence
of degeneration, indicating that at least some part of the calcification of the aortic plaque occurs intracellularly.

Energy dispersive analysis of markedly calcified atherosclerotic lesions revealed a close correlation between calcium and phos-
phorus, suggesting that the material is calcium phosphate. There
was also a close correlation between these two elements and silicon. The role of silicon in the calcification process of the

atheroma is not clear and deserves further investigation.

Grossly, the aortas from the animals of the six weeks regression group were similar to those of the reference group animals.
However, the lesions were less sudanophilic.  On histologic examination, the raised lesions differed from the corresponding reference group lesions by a somewhat thicker fibrous cap, more calcification, a decrease in the number of foam cells, and a marked increase in the number of the macrophage-like cells.  In many instances the latter formed sheets of cells that filled the entire
necrotic portion of the atheromata (Fig. 2-A).

The aortas of the animals from the five-month regression group
showed no flat lesions, but the raised lesions appeared somewhat
flattened, as compared to those of the reference animals, with col-
lapsed and wrinkled centers.  There was a marked decrease in sudanophilia and the vessels were extensively calcified.  On microscopic
examination, there was a marked decrease in the number of foam
cells and a thick fibrous cap was present.  The macrophage-like
cells were much less numerous than at six weeks of regression and
were associated with necrosis.  Necrosis had either disappeared,
being replaced by loose fibrous stroma, or markedly decreased when
compared with the reference or six-seeks regression lesions.  The
residual necrosis was mainly present around calcium deposits which
were more extensive and dense than in the above two groups.

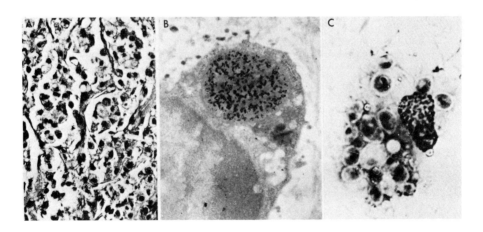

Figure 2.

(A) Illustrates a large accumulation of macrophage-like cells
from a 6 weeks reference lesion of the sequential study.  (B) Ultrastructural histochemical study of non-specific esterase.  Reaction
product is found in lysosome-like structures.  (C) A macrophage
isolated from a lesion has phagocytized numerous yeast particles.

The aortas of the animals from the fourteen-month regression group still showed elevated, slightly sudanophilic and markedly calcified lesions. However, these lesions appeared more flattened than in the other groups. Histologically, there was a virtual absence of foam cells, a further decrease in the size of the necrotic foci and an increase in the thickness and density of the fibrous caps. The macrophage-like cells were present only around the necrotic areas. Calcium deposits appeared more dense than those of the other three groups (Fig. 1-F).

Quantitative assessments showed that there was a significant decrease in both sudanophilia and necrosis in the aortas of the five and fourteen-month regression swine. There was also a gradual decrease in the number of foam cells from the reference lesions to those of the 14-month regression group. The macrophage-like cells were most abundant in the 6-weeks regression lesions; subsequently, they decreased in number. There was no significant change in the ratio of the thickness of the lesion to the average thickness of the media.

Biochemically (Table I), there were no significant differences between the reference group lesions and those of the 6 weeks regression animals, although a considerable numerical drop in free, esterified and total cholesterol was noted at this time. By five months, DNA concentration and esterified cholesterol concentration and synthesis had significantly decreased; esterified and free cholesterol were approximately equal. Collagen synthesis was increased. By fourteen months, synthesis of DNA and total protein had reached control levels, but the concentrations of cholesterol, phospholipids and triglycerides were still substantially elevated. Calcium concentration showed a gradual and significant increase from the reference to the 14-months regression swine.

Histochemical Demonstration of Non-Specific Esterase

Because of the documented prevalence of this enzyme in monocytes and macrophages, we became interested in the use of this enzyme as a marker for quantitating the numbers of macrophages. We studied, histochemically, the localization and pattern of NSE activity at both light and electron microscopic levels during the progression and regression phases of atherosclerosis, using material from the sequential studies experiment. Reaction product was not found in non-lesion areas. All lesions, however, regardless of size and shape, showed non-specific esterase activity to varying degrees. Reaction product was present in macrophages (Fig. 2-B), smooth muscle cells and foam cells in various proportions and configurations, thus negating the value of non-specific esterase as a marker for macrophages. Because of the association of reaction product with atheromata, the data suggest the induction of hydrolytic enzymes in SMC in response to the presence of disease.

Biochemical Assays of Hydrolytic Enzymes

    Results of the biochemical studies of hydrolytic enzyme activi-
ties are presented graphically in Figure 3.  First, it can be seen
that the activities of the three acid hydrolases, cholesteryl ester
hydrolase, β-glucuronidase and collagenolytic activity at pH 3.5,
are each significantly elevated in lesion tissue as compared to the
adjacent non-lesion tissue of animals on high cholesterol diet.  In
addition, the non-lesion tissues of the high cholesterol diet-fed
animals show lower activities of these same enzymes than those of
the non-lesion tissues of mash-fed animals.  In spite of this latter
point, two of these three activities, β-glucuronidase and pH 3.5
collagenolytic are significantly greater in high cholesterol lesion
tissue than in the non-lesion tissue of mash-fed animals.  However,
there is no significant difference seen, in the case of cholesteryl
ester hydrolase, between high cholesterol-fed lesion and mash-fed
non-lesion tissue.

    In contrast to the picture seen with the acid hydrolases, the
pH 7.8 collagenolytic activity of lesions from high cholesterol fed

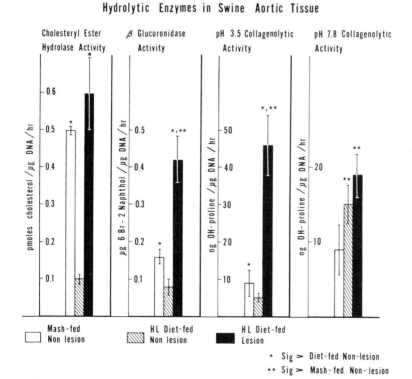

Figure 3.

swine is not significantly greater than that of the adjacent non-
lesion tissue.  Instead, this activity in both types of aortic tissue from the high cholesterol diet-fed animals is significantly
greater than that of the mash-fed non-lesion tissue.

## Study of Phagocytosis

As was stated, we found in our sequential studies a close association between the number of macrophages and necrosis, which suggests a possible role of these cells in the removal of necrotic debris.  By adapting a technique reported by Schaffner (1980) we have
been able to isolate macrophages from well-minced lesion, allow them
to adhere to glass, and demonstrate their ability to phagocytose
yeast by incubating them at 37°C in the presence of Saccharomyces
cerevisiae which has been opsonized by exposure to either fresh
human or fresh swine sera.  The glass adherent cells internalize
varying numbers of yeast cells (Fig. 2-C).

## DISCUSSION

The term "regression" has been used in a variety of contexts
in reports of experimentally-induced atherosclerosis.  In its most
restrictive sense it means a decrease in the thickness or the size
of the lesion.  It has also been applied to the shift in either morphologic or biochemical features toward normal values.  Some aspects of regression are shared with healing, among them the removal
of necrotic material and replacement of some such components with
extracellular substances such as collagen.

We have presented data on the fate of a number of features in
a spectrum of lesions, varying from early proliferative to very advanced, calcified.  The evidence suggests that the occurrence of
"regression" is controlled by at least two factors which interact:
first, the severity of the lesions; second, the degree to which
serum cholesterol levels are lowered.  Further, we have found that
certain features of lesions seem more susceptible to a regression
regimen than others.

Considering the importance of the severity of the lesions in
determination of regressibility, we found that uncomplicated fatty-
proliferative lesions of coronary arteries, and moderately advanced
aortic lesions which showed some complications, such as hemorrhage-
in-plaque and calcium accumulation, did decrease in size after a
period of 12-14 mos of a "regression" diet.  Added evidence that
relatively uncomplicated lesions can be expected to regress is to
be found in the disappearance of essentially all "flat" lesions by
5 mos of regression in the sequential study.  However, the very
severe and extensively calcified lesions, produced by 6 mos of
atherogenic diet and injury in the sequential study, did not de-

crease in size during the 14 mos regression period.  These findings
are in accord with those of other investigators.  Eggen  et al.(1974)
reported regression of fatty streaks, produced in rhesus monkeys by
feeding an atherogenic diet, by shifting the animals to commercial
primate food for 32 and 64 weeks.  They found that the mean extent
of surface involvement with fatty streaks in the aorta and the
brachial, carotid, iliac and femoral arteries was less in the group
sacrificed 32 weeks after diet change as compared to that of the
base line.  There was a further decrease in the second 32 weeks of
diet withdrawal.  Armstrong  et al.(1970) reported that fatty proliferative atherosclerotic plaques in rhesus monkeys on high-cholesterol diet decreased in size significantly when the animals were
shifted to a cholesterol-free diet for 40 months.  They also demonstrated (1972) that during the regression period, there was marked
depletion of both free and esterified cholesterol in the coronary
arteries.  Vesselinovitch  et al.(1976) studied the regression of
moderately advanced atherosclerosis in the rhesus monkey produced
by high cholesterol diet.  They found that after 18 months of diet
withdrawal, the aortas from the regression animals showed about two-
thirds as many lesions which were, on the average, about half as
severe as those on the base-line.  The coronary arteries showed a
similar degree of regression.

The resistance of the very advanced and calcified lesions to
regression was also reported by others:  Prior and Ziegler (1965)
in the rabbit, De Palma  et al.(1972) in the dog and Horlick and
Katz (1949) in chickens.  The latter authors concluded that there
is a limit to the degree of atherosclerotic damage that can be repaired.  However, in our opinion, the question: Will very severe
lesions regress at all, or is there some degree of severity which,
when reached, is irreversible? needs further study.  At present, we
are inclined to believe that the lack of decrease in the size of
lesion in our very severe lesion is due to an insufficient time on
the regression regimen.  It appears there is a possible interaction
between the severity of lesions and the requisite length of time on
a regression regimen required for completion of the regression process.  As pointed out above, flat lesions (fatty streaks) had essentially all disappeared by 5 months of regression.  The moderately
severe lesions resulting from four months' induction had definitely
regressed by 14 mos, with not only a decrease in size, but a remodeling or smoothing of the aortic surface and return of most other
features to normal.  But the 14 mos interval was insufficient to
allow for the very severe lesions, resulting from six months' induction, to decrease in size.  However, the fact that some features
returned to normal during this period is an indication that more
time might have resulted in more regression.  Only experiments in
which comparable lesions are exposed to a regression regimen for
substantially longer times can answer this question definitely.

The importance of the regression dietary regimen's producing

a very low serum cholesterol level is clearly brought out by the
moderate diet-clofibrate study. Here, fatty-proliferative lesions
of the coronary arteries did not decrease in size when the serum
cholesterol levels of the animals were reduced only to 200 mg/dl
and maintained for 12 mos. However, the same diet, achieving cholesterol levels of 100 mg/dl by addition of clofibrate therapy, resulted in a decrease in the thickness of the lesions. This, plus
the fact that the regression of moderately advanced lesions and the
changes toward normalcy that were seen in very advanced lesions were
achieved at serum cholesterol levels at or below 100 mg/dl, indicate
that, in swine, a very low serum cholesterol level is required to
achieve regression.

    Investigators from Winston-Salem studied the effect of a mod-
erate reduction of serum cholesterol on regression in the rhesus
monkey. Monkeys were fed an atherogenic diet for 19 months at which
time a group was sacrificed as a baseline. The remaining animals
were divided into two groups; one group was given a diet designed
to maintain plasma cholesterol concentration at 280-320 mg/dl, and
the other a diet which resulted in plasma cholesterol concentration
of 180-220 mg/dl. Monkeys from each group were sacrificed at 24 and
48 months. At 24 months of regression, gross evaluation of the aortic lesions showed a striking regression of fatty streaks in animals
changed to the 200 mg/dl levels when compared with those from the
baseline or from the 300 mg/dl level. Regression of fibrous plaques
did not occur in either of the regression groups (Bond et al., 1977).
Chemical analysis of the abdominal aortas showed that at 24 months
regression the concentration of total and esterified cholesterol and
of phospholipid had decreased in both regression groups, especially
so in those animals with serum cholesterol levels of 200 mg/dl (Wagner at al.,1980). The reasons underlying the difference between
our findings in the clofibrate study, with essentially no regression
in swine at about 200 mg/dl serum cholesterol, and the regression of
fatty streaks in monkeys with a similar serum cholesterol level cannot be defined at this point. However, it may simply be a function
of severity of the lesion since the lesions we studied are more advanced than fatty streaks. Also, in favor of the above is that, in
their study, fibrous plaques did not regress.

    The differing susceptibilities of various lesion features, ei-
ther morphological or biochemical, to change in the direction of
normalcy in response to a regression diet are interesting. An encouraging point, from the possible prognosis for human lesions, is
the reaction of necrosis, which many believe to be the most sinister
component of the atheroma, with its potential to cause rupture and/
or thrombosis. Regardless of the induction protocol or of the severity of the lesions, necrosis was shown to be susceptible to removal,
or resolution, as a result of a prolonged period of lowered serum
cholesterol levels. It had completely disappeared from the coronary lesions of the clofibrate-treated animals, with their 100 mg/dl

levels, and, by 14 mos, from the moderately severe aortic lesions.
The sequential study added the information that a decrease in the
amount of necrosis was a relatively early event in regression, it
being significantly reduced by 5 mos, and nearly gone by 14 mos, in
spite of the severity of the lesions in this study.  The removal of
necrosis during regression was also reported by Vesselinovitch et
al. (1974, 1976).

Another feature which is very susceptible to change toward normal as a result of a regression regimen is the accumulation of cholesteryl esters.  This is noticeable as early as 6 wks, and becomes
a significant reduction by 5 mos of regression.  The cholesteryl
ester concentration returned to mash control levels by 14 mos of
regression in the case of moderately severe lesions.  However, it
should be noted that this reversion to normal occurred from a lesion
ester cholesterol mean of 11.8 μg/mg dry wt, whereas, when the lesion concentration was higher, 18.8 in the clofibrate study or 74.5
in the sequential study, a return to normal was not achieved in 14
mos.  Rather a level of about one-third that of the reference lesions was the lowest achieved in those experiments.  Perhaps the
ability to clear cholesteryl esters is controlled by the starting
concentration.  The decrease in cholesteryl esters during regression
was also reported in the monkey by Armstrong et al. (1972) and Eggen
et al. (1974) and in the White Carneau pigeon by St. Clair et al.
(1972).

The cellularity is also apparently susceptible to a change in
dietary regimen, since the elevated values in the clofibrate-treated
coronary lesions and in the moderately severe aortic lesions had
reached adjacent non-lesion values by 12 and 14 mos of regression.
This was accompanied by a significant decrease in DNA synthesis in
both cases.  As for the sequential study, DNA concentration in lesions was lower than in control tissues at all time periods, perhaps
reflecting the effects of the vast increase in necrosis and in calcium concentration, since DNA concentration was expressed on a mil-
ligram dry weight basis.  The rate of synthesis of lesion DNA,
though lower at 5 mos than at 6 wks, was still significantly higher
at that time than in the adjacent non-lesion tissue.  But again
by 14 mos, the rate of synthesis had returned to normal levels.

Another consistent finding was the disappearance of foam cells,
which was essentially complete in the coronary lesions of clofibrate-
treated animals, in the moderately severe and in the very severe
aortic lesions by 14 mos.  That the numbers of foam cells are closely related to serum cholesterol levels is suggested by the fact that,
as shown in the sequential studies, they are decreased by about one
half by 6 wks regression, at which time serum cholesterol levels
were nearly the same as mash control values, and half again by 5 mos.
The decrease in foam cells during regression may be the result of a
low proliferative activity and a short life span.  Stary (1974) has

shown by tritiated thymidine autoradiography that there was an increase in the proliferative activity of intimal smooth muscle cells
and foam cells during the hypercholesterolemic state and this returned to the low proliferative activity of control animals during
the regression phase. He also believed (1979) that the foam cells
which are macrophage-derived and have a shorter life span than the
smooth muscle cells, died during the early intervals of lesion regression, while the smooth muscle cells continued to survive.
Hence, the overall numbers of foam cells decreased.

Several investigators have suggested that macrophages are precursors of some or most of the foam cells of the lesion: Stary
(1976), Fowler, et al.(1979), Gerrity, et al.(1979) and Schaffner
(1980). Since we demonstrated that in the early phase of regression
the number of macrophages appeared to increase in parallel with the
decrease in number of foam cells, the possibility that these increased numbers of macrophages represent macrophage-derived foam
cells, which have successfully disposed of their lipid load, must
be considered. An alternative explanation for their presence is the
recruitment of circulating monocytes into the necrotic lesions in
response to some, as yet, unidentified stimulus. Which, if either,
of these possibilities actually occurs in this situation, needs further clarification.

We have also found that macrophages, when present, tend to be
grouped in association with areas of necrosis, and their numbers
fluctuate in parallel with the extent of necrosis. This fact, when
coupled with the demonstration of their capacity to phagocytize
yeast, and with their reported complement of hydrolytic enzymes,
suggests they may be active as effectors of resolution of necrotic
areas.

The results of the biochemical hydrolytic enzyme study are very
interesting. It appears that the atherogenic diet has an overall de-
pressing effect on the three acid hydrolytic activities, cholesteryl
ester hydrolase, $\beta$-glucuronidase and pH 3.5 collagenolytic, since
the activities of the non-lesion tissue of the diet-fed are lower
than those of comparable tissue from mash-fed swine. However, this
depressant effect of the diet is in some fashion abrogated in lesion
tissue, in which the activities of all three are significantly elevated as compared to the adjacent non-lesion tissue. The mechan-
ism(s) controlling this elevated activity in lesion tissues remains
undetermined. In the case of cholesteryl ester hydrolase one might
postulate a substrate induction, since the amount of esterified
cholesterol in lesions can be 20-30 times that of the adjacent non-
lesion tissue. The possibility of substrate induction is not as
attractive as far as $\beta$-glucuronidase and pH 3.5 collagenolytic activities are concerned, because no such striking increase in GAG or
collagen concentrations has been demonstrated in progression lesions.
This divergence among the acid hydrolases emphasizes the fact that
different enzymes may react differently to changes in milieu; their
behavior is not predictable as a group.

Histochemically, the increase in the activity of one acid hydrolase, non-specific esterase, in lesion tissues confirms the general results of the biochemical enzyme studies. It is apparent that this increase in lesion activity can be attributed, not only to the considerable activity seen in macrophages and, to a lesser degree, in foam cells, but also to induction of activity in smooth muscle cells, this activity not being detectable in smooth muscle cells from non-lesion tissue. As in the case of cholesteryl ester hydrolase, here also, substrate induction may play a role. Since one of the many substrates against which non-specific esterase is active is cholesteryl oleate (Morgan et al.,1967), and since we have documented a large increase in cholesteryl ester concentration in the lesions, one can postulate that the same substrate induction is at work for the increased activity of these two enzymes.

One feature of the lesions which did not return to normal in any of the experiments was the accumulation of calcium, although histologically there was some evidence of a decrease in amount of calcium after 12 or 14 mos of regression of lesions of the coronary arteries of the clofibrate-treated animals or the moderately severe aortic lesions. By contrast, both biochemically and histologically, an increase in the amount of calcium throughout the regression period was demonstrated in the very advanced lesion of the sequential studies. The increase in mineralization in this study may be a function of the initial severity of the lesion. Of particular interest are our ultrastructural and energy dispersive studies of calcification which suggest a possible intracellular mechanism and a role of silicon in the calcification process.

A possible cause-effect relationship between increasing amounts of calcium and lack of regression within the 14 mos regression period in the sequential study, and the effect of their high calcium content on the potential for regression of typical advanced human lesions must be considered. Also, the factor(s) triggering this accumulation of calcium, so different from the situation in adjacent non-lesion tissue, needs to be identified and characterized. In favor of the assumption that an increased calcification within the lesion may influence its regression are recent experimental studies which showed that the administration of a calcium antagonist, such as ethane-1-hydroxy-1, 1 diphosphonate, can enhance the regression of the lesions (Wagner et al., 1977; Hollander et al., 1974 and Kramsch & Chan, 1975).

Finally, the goal of our experimental studies of atherosclerosis regression is to identify and characterize the mechanism(s) important in the regression process, with the aim of ultimately being able to enhance these mechanisms and thus improve the potential for the regression of human lesions. We are confining our study to one aspect of regression, the removal of necrotic debris. Our hypothesis is that the most important factors in removal of necrosis

are phagocytosis and the action of hydrolytic enzymes.  So far, we
have shown the presence in lesions of large numbers of macrophages,
demonstrated to be actively phagocytic, in close association with
areas of necrosis, which supports the possible role of phagocytosis.
Our results, both biochemical and histochemical, showing elevated
hydrolytic enzymatic activities associated with lesions, lend cre-
dence to the involvement of hydrolytic enzymes in the resolution of
the atheroma.

REFERENCES

Anitschkow, N. 1933, Experimental atherosclerosis in animals, in:
        "Arteriosclerosis, A Survey of the Problem," E.V. Cowdry,
        ed., Macmillan Co., New York.
Armstrong, M.L. and Megan, M.B., 1972, Lipid depletion in atheroma-
        tous coronary arteries in rhesus monkeys after regression
        diets. Circ Res., 30:675-680.
Armstrong, M.L., Warner, E.D. and Connor, W.E., 1970, Regression of
        coronary atheromatous in rhesus monkeys. Circ Res., 27:59-67.
Aschoff, L., 1924, Lectures in Pathology, in "Atherosclerosis,"
        Chapter 6, Lane Lecture, San Francisco, Hoeber, ed., New York.
Augustyn, J.M., Fritz, K.E., Daoud, A.S., Jarmolych, J. and Lee, K.
        T., 1978, Biochemical effects of moderate diet and clofibrate
        on swine atherosclerosis, Arch Pathol Lab Med., 102:294-297.
Barndt, R., Blankenhorn, D.H., Crawford, D.W. and Brooks, S.H., 1977,
        Regression and progression of early femoral atherosis in
        treated hyperlipoproteinemic patients, Ann Int Med., 86:139-
        146.
Bevans, M., Davidson, J.D. and Kendall, F.E., 1951, Regression of
        lesions in canine arteriosclerosis, Arch Pathol 51:288-292.
Bond, M.G., Bullock, B.C., Lehner, N.D.M. and Clarkson, T.B., 1977,
        Regression of atherosclerosis at plasma cholesterol concen-
        trations achievable in man, in: "Atherosclerosis IV," G.
        Schlettler, Y. Goto, Y. Hata and G. Klose, eds., Springer-
        Verlag, New York.
Bortz, W.M., 1968, Reversibility of atherosclerosis in cholesterol-
        fed rabbits, Circ Res 22:135-139.
Buchwald, H., Rucker, R.D., Moore, R.B. and Varco, R.L., 1980,
        Changes in atherosclerotic lesions following surgical choles-
        terol reduction, in: "Atherosclerosis V," A.M. Gotto, L.C.
        Smith and B. Allen, eds., Springer-Verlag, New York.
Constantinides, P., 1965, Experimental Atherosclerosis, Elsevier
        Publishers, Amsterdam.
Constantinides, P., Booth, J. and Carlson, G., 1960, Production of
        advanced cholesterol atherosclerosis in rabbit. Arch Pathol
        70:712-724.
Daoud, A.S., Jarmolych, J., Augustyn, J.M. and Fritz, K.E., Singh,

J.K. and Lee, K.T., 1976, Regression of advanced atherosclerosis in swine, Arch Pathol Lab Med, 100:372-379.

Daoud, A.S., Jarmolych, J., Augustyn, J.M. and Fritz, K.E., 1981,
Sequential morphologic studies of regression of advanced
atherosclerosis, Arch Pathol Lab Med, 105:233-239.

Delellis, R. and Fishman, W.H., 1965, The variable of pH in the bro-
moindoxylacetate method for the demonstration of esterase,
J Histochem Cytochem, 13:297.

Depalma, R.G., Hubay, C.A. and Insull, W., Jr., 1970, Progression
and regression of experimental atherosclerosis, Surg Gynecol
Obstet, 131:633-647.

DePalma, R.G., Insull, W., Jr. and Bellon, E.M., 1972, Animal models
for the progression and regression of atherosclerosis, Surgery, 72:268-278.

Eggen, D.A., Strong, J.P. and Newman, W.P., III, 1974, Regression of
diet-induced fatty streaks in rhesus monkeys, Lab Invest, 31:
294-301.

Fowler, S., Shio, M.A. and Haley, N.J., 1979, Characterization of
lipid-laden aortic cells from cholesterol-fed rabbits: IV.
Investigation of macrophage-like properties of aortic cell
populations, Lab Invest, 41:372-378.

Fritz, K.E., Augustyn, J.M., Jarmolych, J., Daoud, A.S. and Lee, K.
T., 1976, Regression of advanced atherosclerosis in swine,
Arch Pathol Lab Med, 100:380-385.

Fritz, K.E., Daoud, A.S. and Jarmolych, J., 1980, Non-specific esterase activity during regression of swine aortic atherosclerosis, Artery, 7 (5):352-366.

Fritz, K.E., Augustyn, J.M., Jarmolych, J. and Daoud, A.S., 1981,
Sequential study of biochemical changes during regression of
swine aortic atherosclerotic lesions, Arch Pathol Lab Med,
105:240-246.

Gerrity, R.G., Naito, H.K. and Richardson, M., 1979, Dietary induced
atherogenesis in swine, Am J Pathol, 95:775-792.

Goldbarg, J.A., Pineda, E.P., Banks, B.M. and Rutenberg, A.N., 1959,
A method for the colorimetric determination of β-glucuroni-
in urine, serum and tissue; assay of enzymatic activity in
health and disease, Gastroenterology, 36:193-201.

Hollander, W., McCombs, H.L., Franzblau, C., Kirkpatrick, B. and
Schmid, K., 1974, Influence of the anticalcifying agent,
ethane-1-hydroxy-1, 1-diphosphonate (EHDP) on pre-established
atheromata in rabbits. Circ, 50:3.

Horlick, L. and Katz, L.N., 1949, Retrogression of atherosclerotic
lesions on cessation of cholesterol feeding in the chick,
J Lab Med, 34:1427-1442.

Jarmolych, J., Daoud, A.S., Fritz, K.E., Augustyn, J.M., Singh, J.K.
and Kim, D.N., 1978, Morphologic effects of moderate diet and
clofibrate on swine atherosclerosis, Arch Pathol Lab Med,
102:289-293.

Kim, K.M., 1976, Calcification of matrix vesicles in human aortic
valve and aortic media, Fed Proc, 35:156.

Kim, K.M. and Trump, B.F., 1975, Amorphous calcium precipitations in human aortic valve, Calcif Tiss Res, 18:155.

Kothari, H.V., Miller, B.F. and Kritchevsky, D., 1973, Aortic cholesterol esterase: characteristics of normal and rabbit enzyme, Biochem Biophys Acta, 296:446-454.

Kramsch, D.M. and Chan, C.T., 1975, Effects of ethane-hydroxy-diphosphonate (EHDP) and n-acetyl-n-methyl-colchicine (Colcemid) on progression and regression of experimental atherosclerosis, Fed Proc, 34:235.

Malmros, H., 1950, The relation of nutrition to health. A statistical study of the effect of the war-time on arteriosclerosis, cardiosclerosis, tuberculosis and diabetes, Acta Med Scand, 246:137-153.

McMillan, G.C., Horlick, L. and Duff, G.L., 1955, Cholesterol content of aorta in relation to severity of atherosclerosis, Arch Path, 59:285.

Morgan, R.G.H., Barrowman, J., Filipek-Wender, H. and Borgstrom, B., 1967, The lipolytic enzymes of rat pancreatic juice, Biochem Biophys Acta, 146:314-316.

Pick, R., Stamler, J. and Rodbard, S., 1952, Estrogen-induced regression of coronary atherosclerosis in cholesterol-fed chicks, Circ, 6:858-861.

Prior, J.T. and Ziegler, D.D., 1965, Regression of experimental atherosclerosis, Arch Pathol, 80:50-57.

St. Clair, R.W., Clarkson, T.B. and Lofland, H.B., 1972, Effects of regression of atherosclerotic lesions on the content and esterification of cholesterol by cell-free preparations of pigeon aorta, Circ Res, 31:664-671.

Schaffner, T., Taylor, K. and Bartucci, E.J., 1980, Arterial foam cells with distinctive immunomorphologic and histochemical features of macrophages, Am J Pathol, 100:57-80.

Stary, H.C., 1974, Cell proliferation and ultrastructural changes in regressing atherosclerotic lesions after reduction of serum cholesterol, in: "Atherosclerosis III," G. Schlettler and A. Weizel, eds., Springer-Verlag, New York

Stary, H.C., 1976, Coronary artery fine structure in rhesus monkeys: The early atherosclerotic lesion and its progression, Primates Med, 9:359-395.

Stary. H.C., 1979, Regression of atherosclerosis in primates, Virchows Arch A Path Anat and Histol, 383:117-134.

Strom, A. and Jensen, R.A., 1951, Mortality from circulatory disease in Norway 1940-1945, Lancet, 1:126.

Takano, T., Black, W.J., Peters, T.J. and DeDuer, C., 1974, Assay, kinetics, and lysosomal localization of an acid cholesteryl esterase in aortic rabbit smooth muscle cells, J Biol Chem, 249:6732-6737.

Vesselinovitch, D., Wissler, R.W., Hughes, R. and Borensztajn, J., 1976, Reversal of advanced atherosclerosis in rhesus monkeys, Atherosclerosis, 23:155-176.

Vesselinovitch, D., Wissler, R.W., Fisher-Dzoga, K., Hughes, R. and

Dubien, L. 1974, Regression of atherosclerosis in rabbits. Part 1. Treatment with low-fat diet, hyperoxia and hypo-lipidemic agents. Atherosclerosis 19:259-275.

Wagner, W.D., Clarkson, T.B. and Foster, J., 1977, Contrasting effects of ethane-1-hydroxy-1, 1-diphosphonate (EHDP) on the regression of two types of dietary-induced atherosclerosis, Atherosclerosis, 27:419-435.

Wagner, W.D., St. Clair, R.W. and Clarkson, T.B., 1980, A study of atherosclerosis regression in macaca mulatta. II. Chemical changes in arteries from animals with atherosclerosis induced for 19 months then regressed for 24 months at plasma choles-terol concentrations of 300 or 200 mg/dl, Exp Molec Pathol, 32:162-174.

Wanscher, O., Clemmesen, J. and Nielsen, A., 1951, Negative correla-tion between atherosclerosis and carcinoma, Brit J Cancer, 5:172.

Wilens, S.L., 1947, Resorption of arterial atheromatic deposits in wasting disease, Am J Path, 23:273.

Yam, L.T., Li, C.Y. and Crosby, W.H., 1971, Cytochemical identifi-cation of monocytes and granulocytes, Amer J Clin Pathol, 55:283-290.

# REGRESSION OF CORONARY ATHEROSCLEROSIS

# IN MAN

N.B. Myant

Medical Research Council Lipid Metabolism Unit
Hammersmith Hospital
London W12 0HS, U.K.

## INTRODUCTION

### Regression of Experimental Atherosclerosis

There is abundant evidence that it is possible to bring about some degree of regression of experimentally-induced atherosclerosis of the coronary arteries in animals (see Armstrong, 1976, for review). Much of the published work on regression of atheroscler-osis induced in animals by diets, with or without concomitant injury to the arterial walls, has been concerned with the reversal of lesions that bear more resemblance to fatty streaks than to the fully developed lesions associated with ischaemic heart disease in man. However, there can be no doubt that lesions in the coronary arteries, closely resembling the naturally-occurring human athero-matous lesion, can be induced in monkeys by the prolonged feeding of cholesterol-rich diets, and that withdrawal of the dietary regimen may result in partial regression of the lesions, with widening of the lumen, loss of intimal lipid and, possibly, a decrease in the amount of collagen in the arterial wall (Armstrong et al., 1970; Vesselinovitch et al., 1976; Stary et al., 1977). A survey of the relevant literature suggests that the time taken to bring about regression of experimentally-induced atherosclerosis by withdrawal of the atherogenic regimen is at least as long as the time taken to induce the atherosclerosis (Vesselinovitch and Wissler, 1977), and that in order to induce significant regression in monkeys the plasma cholesterol concentration must be reduced to less than 200 mg/100 ml throughout the regression period (Bond et al., 1977).

## Relevance to Regression of Human Coronary Atherosclerosis

These observations on experimental animals suggest that it should be possible to bring about partial regression of naturally-occurring atherosclerosis of the coronary arteries in man by prolonged and substantial reduction of the plasma cholesterol concentration.   This expectation is, of course, based on the tacit assumption that the pathology of the human lesions is broadly similar to that of the diet-induced lesions in animals.   However, it is possible that coronary atherosclerosis associated with hypertension or cigarette smoking, or with causal factors not yet identified, differs in some subtle way from coronary atherosclerosis in which hypercholesterolaemia is the main cause.   In this case it would not be surprising if prolonged reduction of the plasma cholesterol concentration turned out to be more effective in inducing regression of lesions in people who are hypercholesterolaemic than in those who have never had a raised plasma cholesterol level.   This point is worth bearing in mind in view of the frequent occurrence of ischaemic heart disease in people whose plasma cholesterol concentration is within the statistically normal range.

EVIDENCE FOR REGRESSION IN MAN

## Indirect Evidence

Much of the available evidence for regression of coronary atherosclerosis in man is indirect or controversial.   It has often been noted that the incidence of coronary atherosclerosis in adult human subjects who have died after a limited period of severe malnutrition is much lower than that in age-matched control subjects from the same population (for references, see Armstrong, 1976). This has been taken as circumstantial evidence for regression of lesions presumed to have been present before the period of malnutrition.   The possible success of some primary or secondary prevention trials in which a fatal or non-fatal heart attack is taken as the end point also suggests that coronary atherosclerosis can be reversed or caused to progress more slowly.   However, trials in which the end point is a clinical occurrence require very large numbers of subjects if the number of events is to be sufficient for statistical analysis.   Furthermore, such trials do not provide any evidence as to the state of the coronary arteries in the treated and control populations during the course of the trial.   It is possible, for example, that a reduction in the incidence of heart attacks as a result of some form of intervention is due to an effect on the vessel-wall thrombosis responsible for the final occlusion, rather than to reversal or lack of progression of the underlying atherosclerotic process.   An alternative approach is to use serial angiography in small populations of high-risk subjects given intensive treatment to counteract the risk. Three such tests of the regression hypothesis in small groups of hypercholesterolaemic subjects, most of whom had FH[*], will be discussed in this review.

## Partial Ileal Bypass

Surgical removal or bypass of a substantial segment of the ileum has long been known to cause a marked fall in the plasma cholesterol concentration, an effect that is probably due to interference with the reabsorption of bile salts from the ileum, leading to stimulation of the conversion of hepatic cholesterol into bile acids. Buchwald (1964) has exploited this effect as a means of lowering the plasma cholesterol concentration in patients with essential hypercholesterolaemia. Having established that bypass of the distal 200 cm of the ileum would bring about a fall of 40% or more in the plasma cholesterol level in hyperlipidaemic subjects, Buchwald and coworkers (Buchwald et al., 1974) initiated a trial of the effects of the operation on the clinical course and appearance of coronary angiograms in a group of patients with primary type II hypercholesterolaemia, most of whom were probably suffering from FH. In some of these patients regression or disappearance of xanthelasmas and of xanthomas of the skin and tendons was observed. There was also a decrease in the frequency and severity of angina pectoris in more than half the patients treated, with complete remission of symptoms in about a quarter. Coronary angiography, carried out before and 2 years after the operation in 22 patients, showed evidence suggestive of increased luminal diameter in two and a decrease in the size of plaques in three; in one of these, recanalization of an occluded left anterior descending coronary artery was noted. In the remaining 17 patients who underwent serial angiography twelve showed no change and five showed progression or a new occlusion.

## Diet Combined with a Bile-Acid Sequestrant

Colestipol, a plasma-cholesterol-lowering drug, is an unabsorbable anion exchange resin that binds bile salts in the intestine and thus prevents their reabsorption. As a means of treating hypercholesterolaemia it is therefore the medical equivalent of an operation for partial ileal bypass. In a trial analogous to that of Buchwald et al. (1974), Kuo et al. (1979) have studied the effect of prolonged treatment with colestipol and a low-fat diet on coronary atherosclerosis in a group of hypercholesterolaemic patients, most of whom appear to have had FH in the heterozygous form. The

---

[*]Abbreviations used are:- FH, familial hypercholesterolaemia; HDL, high-density lipoprotein; LDL, low-density lipoprotein.

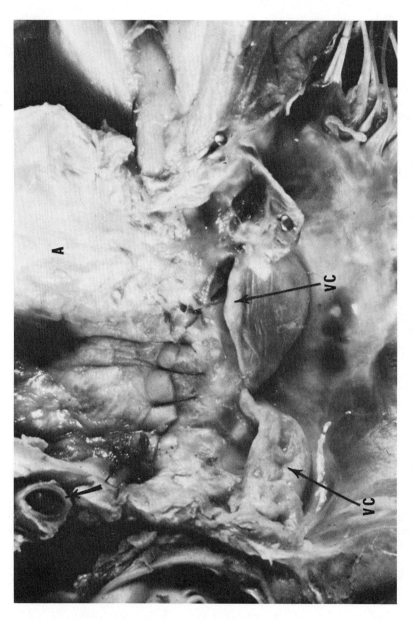

Fig. 1.   Aortic root and valve cusps from the heart of a homozygous FH patient (PA of Table 1). The luminal surface of the aortic root (A) and parts of the valve cusps (VC) are infiltrated with xanthomatous lipid.   Upper arrow shows the cut end of a by-pass tube inserted shortly before the patient died.   (From Myant, 1981.)

combination of diet and drug brought about a mean fall of 34% in plasma total cholesterol concentration and of 43% in LDL-cholesterol concentration, with no significant change in HDL-cholesterol concentration. The net effect in the group as a whole was a significant increase in the HDL/LDL cholesterol ratio. In 12 patients, coronary angiograms were obtained before and 3 to 4 years after the beginning of treatment. In the 8 patients in whom there was a substantial fall in plasma LDL-cholesterol concentration and a fall in total cholesterol level to a mean value of 270 mg/100 ml, there was no change in the angiographic appearance of the coronary arteries. In the other four, in whom the hypercholesterolaemia was not controlled, angiography showed progression of the coronary atherosclerosis, with complete occlusion of a coronary vessel in three patients.

Repeated Plasma Exchange

For the purpose of testing for the possible reversibility of coronary atherosclerosis in man, potentially the most suitable trial population would be a group of patients with a well-defined disease in which coronary atherosclerosis is invariably and rapidly progressive in the absence of treatment. A condition that fulfills these criteria is FH in the homozygous form or in its most severe heterozygous form. In homozygous FH, atherosclerosis progresses rapidly in the coronary arteries and aortic root (Fig. 1), leading to death from ischaemic heart disease in the second or third decade, few patients surviving beyond the mid-twenties; in the more severely hypercholesterolaemic males with heterozygous FH, the risk of premature coronary heart disease is only a little less than that in homozygotes (see Myant, 1981). However, a major drawback to using these patients to test the regression hypothesis lies in their marked resistance to any attempt to lower the plasma cholesterol level by diet or drugs. For example, treatment with maximal doses of cholestyramine, a drug that is very effective in lowering the plasma cholesterol level in FH heterozygotes with moderate hypercholesterolaemia, has essentially no effect in FH homozygotes (Moutafis et al., 1977). However, the relatively recent development of a method for replacing the patient's plasma with a cholesterol-free substitute by means of a continuous-flow cell separator has made it possible to overcome this difficulty.

Since 1974, Thompson and coworkers (Thompson et al., 1975, 1980) have been studying the feasibility and effectiveness of repeated plasma exchanges in a small group of FH patients, the majority of whom were homozygotes. We have shown that it is possible to exchange 2-4 litres of the patient's plasma with plasma protein fraction at fortnightly intervals on an outpatient basis for up to 5 years, without side-effects and with the minimum of inconvenience to the patient.

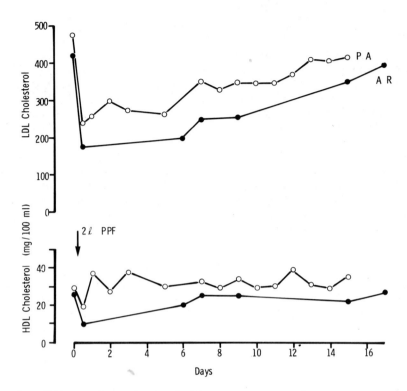

Fig. 2.   Effect of a single 2-litre exchange with plasma protein
          fraction (PPF) on plasma LDL- and HDL-cholesterol concen-
          tration in 2 patients with homozygous FH (PA and AR of
          Table 1).    (From Thompson et al., 1975.)


        Changes in plasma cholesterol concentration.    During each
exchange there is a rapid fall in plasma total and LDL cholesterol
concentration, followed by a slow return to the pre-exchange level
during the subsequent 2 weeks (Fig. 2), the rate of rise being more
rapid in homozygotes than in heterozygotes.    The mean plasma cholesterol concentration between successive exchanges may be expressed
as the area under the curve between exchanges, divided by the time
interval.    Fig. 3 shows the mean plasma cholesterol levels in two
homozygotes who underwent repeated plasma exchange.    As would be
expected, the effect of a series of exchanges on the cholesterol
level is determined mainly by the volume of plasma exchanged in
relation to the patient's plasma volume, and the frequency of
exchanges.    In DL, it was possible to reduce the mean level from an
initial value of 610 mg/100 ml to well below 300 mg/100 ml by weekly
exchanges of 3.2 litres combined with nicotinic acid by mouth, the
effect of this drug being to diminish the rate of rise of the plasma
cholesterol level after each exchange.    Fig. 4 shows the mean
plasma cholesterol levels in two FH heterozygotes during a course of

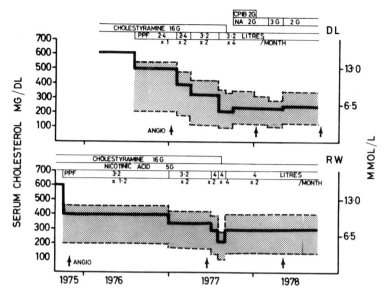

Fig. 3   Effect of plasma exchanges on the maximum, minimum and
mean (solid line) serum cholesterol concentration in 2
FH homozygotes.  CPIB, clofibrate; NA, nicotinic acid;
PPF, plasma protein fraction.  (From Thompson et al.,
1980.)

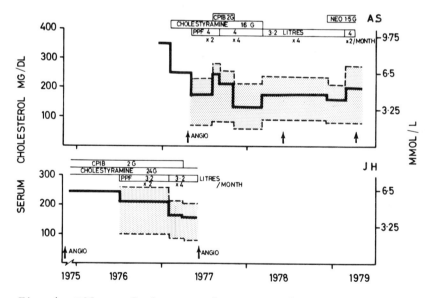

Fig. 4   Effect of plasma exchanges on the mean, maximum and
minimum serum cholesterol concentration in 2 FH heterozygotes.  Details are the same as in Fig. 3.

repeated plasma exchange.    In both patients, mean values of less
than 200 mg/100 ml were achieved.    In Table 1 the plasma cholesterol
levels achieved during periods of repeated plasma exchange are shown
for four homozygotes, including the two shown in Fig. 3, and for the
two heterozygotes shown in Fig. 4.

Comparable effects of plasma exchange on the plasma cholesterol
in FH homozygotes have been reported by others (Berger et al., 1978;
King et al., 1980; Stein et al., 1981).    Simons et al. (1978) have
also used repeated plasma exchange in the treatment of FH heterozygotes.    In their hands the effect of plasma exchange on the plasma
cholesterol was no greater than that of standard medical treatment,
but this may have been due to their carrying out the exchanges at
monthly rather than fortnightly intervals.

Angiography.    To assess the effect of the sustained reduction
in plasma cholesterol level on the state of the coronary arteries
and aortic root, serial cineangiographic studies of the aorta and
coronary arteries were carried out, with measurement of the
ventriculo-aortic systolic pressure gradient.    Paired frames from
pre- and post-exchange films, matched for anatomical position and
phase of the cardiac cycle, were examined by an independent "blind"
observer (Thompson et al., 1980).

In all the homozygotes examined initially, aortography
showed the characteristic narrowing and irregularity of the
proximal aorta (Fig. 5) previously noted by Stanley et al.
(1965) in a child with homozygous FH and described more recently
in seven FH homozygotes investigated at Hammersmith Hospital

Table 1.    Plasma Cholesterol Concentration in 6 FH Patients Before
and During a Period of Repeated Plasma Exchange

| Patient | Age | Initial Cholesterol (mg/100 ml) | Plasma Exchanges | | | Mean Cholesterol Throughout Exchanges (mg/100 ml) |
|---|---|---|---|---|---|---|
| | | | Number | Duration (months) | Volume (litres) | |
| PA (F) | 23 | 812 | 24 | 22 | 2–2.4 | 518 |
| AR (F) | 26 | 625 | 9 | 10 | 2–2.4 | 440 |
| RW (M) | 25 | 605 | 66[a] | 38 | 3.2–4 | 336 |
| DL (M) | 15 | 610 | 78[a] | 28 | 2.4–3.2 | 325 |
| JH (M) | 31 | 258 | 33 | 12 | 3.2 | 189 |
| AS (M) | 47 | 356 | 72 | 23 | 3.2–4 | 169 |

[a]Each of these patients has now (September 1981) had more than 120
exchanges.    PA, AR, RW and DL are homozygotes;    JH and AS are
heterozygotes.

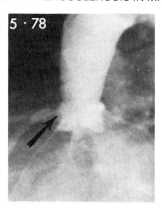

Fig. 5. Aortogram from a 25-year-old man (RW) with FH in the homozygous form, showing the characteristic narrowing and irregularity of the lumen of the aortic root due to infiltration with xanthomatous lipid. Note the right coronary stricture shown by the arrow. (From Thompson et al., 1980.)

(Allen et al., 1980). The underlying lesion responsible for the peculiar angiographic outline shown in Fig. 5 is a gross thickening of the intima of the root of the aorta and of the aortic valve cusps and sinuses of Valsalva, due to atheromatous deposits. In all four homozygotes there was also narrowing of one or both coronary ostia, with narrowing and irregularity of the coronary arteries, particularly in their proximal portions. In the two heterozygotes the pre-exchange aortograms were normal, but angiography showed bilateral atheromatous involvement of coronary arteries in both patients.

Long-term effects of plasma exchange. After 2 to 3 years of repeated plasma exchange combined with nicotinic acid, there was almost complete resolution of the cutaneous xanthomas in RW and DL, and a marked reduction in the size of their tendon xanthomas. There was no change in the appearance of the xanthomas in PA and AR.

The angiographic studies showed decreased mobility of the aortic valve cusps in AR, but the appearances of the supravalvular portion of the aorta and of the coronary vessels did not change during nearly 3 years of plasma exchange in RW and DL. As a quantitative index of the extent of narrowing of the aortic root, the ratio of the diameter of the narrowest portion to that of the adjacent unaffected segment was measured. No change was observed in AR, RW and DL, the three patients in whom pre- and post-exchange observations were made (Table 2). The peak systolic ventriculo-aortic gradient remained unchanged in RW and DL, but there were substantial increases in PA and AR (Table 2), indicative of progressive involvement of the valve cusps by atheroma or fibrosis.

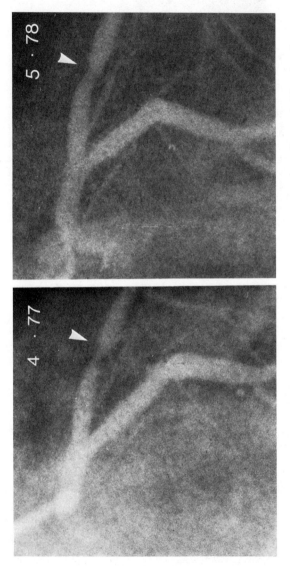

Fig. 6.   Coronary angiogram from a heterozygous FH patient (AS) showing a stricture of the anterior descending branch of the left coronary artery (arrows) before (left frame) and after (right frame) plasma exchange for 13 months.   (From Thompson et al., 1980.)

Table 2.   Left Ventriculo-Aortic Peak Systolic Gradients and
           Aortographic Appearances in 4 Homozygous FH Patients
           Undergoing Plasma Exchange

| Patient | Date of Angiograms | Gradient (mm Hg) | Aortic Ratio[a] |
|---------|--------------------|-------------------|------------------|
| PA      | 9/74               | 35                | –                |
|         | 11/76              | 75                | –                |
| AR      | 1/75               | 34                | 0.59             |
|         | 11/78              | 130               | 0.58             |
| RW      | 10/75              | 40                | 0.73             |
|         | 5/78               | 50                | 0.71             |
| DL      | 1/77               | 19                | 0.67             |
|         | 10/78              | 20                | 0.64             |

[a]Expressed as the ratio: $\dfrac{\text{Diameter of narrowed lumen}}{\text{Diameter of adjacent normal lumen}}$
   (From Thompson et al., 1980.)

In JH the appearance of the coronary arteries was unchanged after plasma exchange for a year, but in AS there was an apparent increase in diameter at the site of a stricture of the anterior descending limb of the left coronary artery (Fig. 6).

Discussion of Results

None of these trials provides conclusive evidence that a sustained fall in plasma cholesterol concentration has a favourable effect on the atherosclerotic lesions in the coronary arteries and basal aorta in FH.   In none of the 3 studies was there a group of untreated subjects comparable with those given the treatment. Furthermore, however carefully the angiographic procedures are standardized in successive investigations, it is very difficult to detect small differences in luminal diameter or plaque size at intervals of a year or longer.   Nevertheless, the results of the 3 trials considered together are distinctly encouraging.   The normal sequence of events in human coronary atherosclerosis seems to be progression of the lesions.   Thus, Bemis et al. (1973) noted progression in 52% of patients with coronary artery disease examined by angiography at an average interval of 2 years, and Kimbiris et al. (1974) observed progression in 68.5% of patients during a similar interval.   In the 3 trials discussed above, the angiographic appearance of the coronary arteries showed no detectable change over periods measured in years in most of the patients in whom a

significant reduction in plasma cholesterol level was achieved.
This suggests very strongly that the progress of coronary atherosclerosis can be halted in hypercholesterolaemic patients, an
impression that is reinforced by our own observations on the four FH
homozygotes treated by plasma exchange.  In the two in whom the mean
plasma cholesterol level was reduced to less than 300 mg/100 ml
(with, of course, much greater reductions for short periods immediately after each exchange) there was no detectable change in the
coronary arteries, aortic root or ventriculo-aortic pressure gradient
during a 2 to 3 year period.  On the other hand, in PA and AR, in
whom the mean fall in plasma cholesterol level was much less, aortic
stenosis progressed.

In the ileal-bypass and plasma-exchange studies there was
evidence suggestive of true regression in several of the FH heterozygotes.  This was particularly striking in AS, in the plasma-
exchange study, and in the patient in whom there was recanalization
of an occluded coronary artery after ileal bypass.  However, it
should be noted that spontaneous resolution of an occluded coronary
artery has been recorded, though not in FH (Landmann et al., 1976).

Finally, it should be borne in mind that even if regression of
coronary atherosclerosis could be demonstrated unequivocally in FH,
this would not necessarily be relevant to the question of the
reversibility of atherosclerosis in the general population.  Although
the lesions in FH heterozygotes are indistinguishable in their
distribution and morphology from those in people who do not carry
the FH gene, atherosclerosis due predominantly to a life-long
increase in plasma LDL concentration may differ at the cellular or
subcellular level from that due to a multiplicity of causes.  These
considerations apply with greater force to homozygous FH, in which
the lesions have an abnormal preponderance of intracellular lipid
and an atypical distribution.

REFERENCES

Allen, J. M., Thompson, G. R., Myant, N. B., Steiner, R., and Oakley,
      C. M., 1980, Cardiovascular complications of homozygous
      familial hypercholesterolaemia, Brit. Heart J., 44:361.
Armstrong, M. L., 1976, Regression of atherosclerosis, in:
      "Atherosclerosis Review," R. Paoletti, and A. M. Gotto, ed.,
      Raven Press, New York.
Armstrong, M. L., Warner, E. D., and Connor, W. E., 1970, Regression
      of coronary atheromatosis in rhesus monkeys, Circulation
      Res., 27:59.
Bemis, C. E., Gorlin, R., Kemp, H. G., and Herman, M. V., 1973,
      Progression of coronary artery disease. A clinical arterio-
      graphic study, Circulation, 47:455.
Berger, G. M. B., Miller, J. L., Bonnici, F., Joffe, H. S., and
      Dubovsky, D. W., 1978, Continuous flow plasma exchange in the

treatment of homozygous familial hypercholesterolemia,
Am. J. Med., 65:243.

Bond, M. G., Bullock, B. C., Lehner, N. D. M., and Clarkson, T. B.,
1977, Regression of atherosclerosis at plasma concentrations
available to man, in: "Atherosclerisis IV," G. Schettler,
Y. Goto, Y. Hata, and G. Klose, ed., Springer-Verlag, Berlin.

Buchwald, H., 1964, Lowering of cholesterol absorption and blood
levels by ileal exclusion. Experimental basis and preliminary
clinical report, Circulation, 29:713.

Buchwald, H., Moore, R. B., and Varco, R. L., 1974, Surgical treatment of hyperlipidemia, Circulation, 49, Suppl. I:I-1.

Kimbiris, D., Lavine, P., van den Broek, H., Najmi, M., and Likoff,
W., 1974, Devolutionary pattern of coronary atherosclerosis
in patients with angina pectoris. Coronary angiographic
studies, Am. J. Cardiol., 33:7.

King, M. E. E., Breslow, J. L., and Lees, R. W., 1980, Plasma-
exchange therapy of homozygous familial hypercholesterolemia,
New Engl. J. Med., 302:1457.

Kuo, P. T., Hayase, K., Kostis, J. B., and Moreyra, A. E., 1979,
Use of combined diet and colestipol in long-term (7-7½ years)
treatment of patients with type II hyperlipoproteinemia,
Circulation, 59:199.

Landmann, J., Kolsters, W., and Bruschke, A. V. G., 1976, Regression
of coronary artery obstructions demonstrated by coronary
arteriography, Eur. J. Cardiol., 4:475.

Moutafis, C. D., Simons, L. A., Myant, N. B., Adams, P. W., and Wynn,
V., 1977, The effect of cholestyramine on the faecal excretion
of bile acids and neutral steroids in familial hypercholesterolaemia, Atherosclerosis, 26:329.

Myant, N. B., 1981, "The Biology of Cholesterol and Related
Steroids," Heinemann Medical Books, London.

Simons, L. A., Gibson, J. C., Isbister, J. P., and Biggs, J. C.,
1978, The effects of plasma exchange on cholesterol
metabolism, Atherosclerosis, 31:195.

Stanley, P., Chartrand, C., and Davignon, A., 1965, Acquired aortic
stenosis in a twelve-year-old girl with xanthomatosis, New
Engl. J. Med., 273:1378.

Stary, H. C., Eggen, D. A., and Strong, J. P., 1977, The mechanism
of atherosclerosis regression, in: "Atherosclerosis IV,"
G. Schettler, Y. Goto, Y. Hata, and G. Klose, ed., Springer-
Verlag, Berlin.

Stein, E. A., Glueck, C. J., Wesselman, A., Owens, E. R., Nichols,
S., and Vink, P., 1981, Repetitive intermittent flow plasma
exchange in patients with severe hypercholesterolemia,
Atherosclerosis, 38:149.

Thompson, G. R., Lowenthal, R., and Myant, N. B., 1975, Plasma exchange in the management of homozygous familial hypercholesterolaemic, Lancet, 1:1208.

Thompson, G. R., Myant, N. B., Kilpatrick, D., Oakley, C. M.,
Raphael, M. J., and Steiner, R. E., 1980, Assessment of long-

term plasma exchange for familial hypercholesterolaemia,
Brit. Heart J., 43:680.

Vesselinovitch, D., and Wissler, R. W., 1977, Requirement for
regression studies in animal models, in: "Atherosclerosis IV,"
G. Schettler, Y. Goto, Y. Hata, and G. Klose, ed., Springer-
Verlag, Berlin.

Vesselinovitch, D., Wissler, R. W., Hughes, R., and Borensztajn, J.
1976, Reversal of advanced atherosclerosis in rhesus monkeys.
Part 1. Light-microscopic studies, Atherosclerosis, 23:155.

INDEX